Ilaria Capua

CIRCULAR HEALTH

Empowering the
One Health Revolution

Foreword by
Louise O. Fresco

Translation: Lucy Lennon
Copyediting: Jill Connelly, Cristina Saccuman
Typesetting: Alberto Bellanti
Cover: Cristina Bernasconi

The background image on the cover is taken from Isidorus Hispalensis, *De Natura Rerum*, Cod. 83-II, fol. 131v (detail), manuscript preserved at Koeln, Erzbischoefliche Dioezesan- und Dombibliothek/Cologne, Library of the Cathedral and of the Archdiocese. We thank them for granting us permission to reproduce the image.

EGEA S.p.A.
Via Salasco, 5 - 20136 Milano
Tel. 02/5836.5751 – Fax 02/5836.5753
egea.edizioni@unibocconi.it – www.egeaeditore.it

First edition: July 2020

ISBN Domestic Edition 978-88-99902-60-5
ISBN International Edition 978-88-85486-94-2
ISBN Digital International Edition 978-88-31322-22-5
ISBN Digital Domestic Edition 978-88-238-1931-3

To the survivors of COVID-19
and the NLs of yesterday, today, and tomorrow

You will never discover the impossible,
unless you are prepared to find it.
(Anonymous)

Contents

Foreword

by *Louise O. Fresco*

This is a book about science, infectious diseases in particular, but also about how science and politics intertwine and the journey of a single scientist to disentangle them. Virology has become so popular since the outbreak of the Covid-19 pandemic that nearly everybody claims to be a virologist these days. It is, of course, a serious and complex science.

I first met the author, Professor Ilaria Capua, in Rome when I was working at FAO, at the time of the 2005 H5N1 avian influenza epidemic. Some of her most important scientific work was conducted then as she characterized viruses for the first time and developed vaccination strategies to assist in their control. In this book she takes us on a journey to understand the intricacies and unexpected aspects of the discovery of certain infectious diseases and, indirectly, shows us how difficult it is to act in the case of an unknown zoonotic virus.

This is also a book about how science is conducted. Science does not exist in isolation: its context is always political and societal. Societies expect and desire outcomes, and occasionally, when the outcomes are not easily understood or do not fit political framing, damage and even drama may occur. While the context here is mostly in the past, the lessons for today's world are clear. It is interdisciplinarity which makes the big difference.

But the ultimate message of this book is to consider health as resource that needs to be managed and empowered. Health of humans, animals, plants and the environment are interconnected and interdependent and this means acknowledging a full understanding of the system. The interconnected ecological and human systems in which we live have allowed wild animals, such as bats or migratory birds, to carry viruses that threaten domestic animals and also human beings, Covid-19 being just last on the list. Urban, rural, and wild ecosystems are connected all over the earth through multiple drivers such as water, waste and food systems.

The staggering increase in urbanization and mobility of people and goods all contribute to the risk of emerging and re-emerging infectious diseases. And chronic diseases, which still account for the vast majority of human mortality, may play a role in aggravating the risks to vulnerable groups. This setting, in combination with the as yet unknown effects of climate change on disease vectors, forces us to take an integrated and interdisciplinary approach. Although she started as a veterinary virologist, Ilaria reaches beyond the conventional subject boundaries and makes a convincing case for a broader view of health. She calls it Circular Health, because it is circular systems that represent a central and vital connection hub between humans and nature.

Perhaps the most important contribution of the book is its insistence on the sharing of knowledge and data now that we are immersed in the big data environment. Ilaria's scientific intuition back in 2006 on sharing genetic sequences in the face of the H5N1 crisis seems obvious today in the midst of the 2020 pandemic. My favorite axioma is that knowledge is the only truly sustainable resource: using and sharing it never exhausts it, and in fact is the road to its multiplication. The conviction that sharing is essential today finds additional grounds as artificial intelligence and next generation computing become among of the tools of the future.

This book invites us to stretch our imagination by using lateral thinking and data driven science to co-advance the health of humans, animals, plants and the environment in a sustainable and integrated manner. Advancing health as a system by exploiting the digital revolution may well be one of the leading paradigm shifts which can help our species, *Homo sapiens*, to address and intervene on some of the huge challenges that lie ahead.

Wageningen, July 2020

-7   This Book Is Not About COVID-19

COVID-19 and its dramatic consequences are just one of the examples of what this book is about.

Let's rewind to early 2019, when I started writing Circular Health. The undeniable reality of climate change was one of the main causes of tension among governments. This was mainly due to a significant polarization of opinions over the possibility that current extreme weather events have their origins in human-related activities. The polarizing question is whether melting ice caps, bleaching coral reefs and raging wildfires in Australia, the Amazon and California are part of a natural cycle or not. It would seem more logical to enact measures to counteract rising temperatures regardless of the resultant global warming being a transitory event or a more permanent trend. Whatever the origins of the problem – we should strive to regain the natural equilibrium. This is only one of the global challenges which is interconnected with many others. Another example? The global freshwater crisis. Fire and water.

The natural interconnections between fire, water, and earth in 2020 clash violently with the nutritional requirements of exploding demographics in under-resourced countries. We are all aware that to feed the world we will need to rebalance agricultural production. Rising sea levels are expected to completely transform our coastlines. What's more, overfishing and pollution are making our oceans lose their balance and biodiversity. But this is all bad enough as it stands, without considering the fourth element: air. Today, our source of oxygen is polluted to unbelievable levels. And if this air pollution accelerates, it will become even more powerful and immensely destructive.

At the dawn of 2020, we have suddenly found ourselves at the mercy of a virtually unknown virus which erupted in the heart of a megacity that most of us had never even heard of before. But what happened inside the beating heart of Wuhan, China? The truth is that we don't know yet, but the evidence we have is that a bat coronavirus acquired a component of another coronavirus which, as we go to press, is believed to have originated from a pangolin. Whether or not this part of the story is true is rather irrelevant – but what is relevant is that we've created the perfect environment for pandemic pathogens to be generated and sustained in certain host populations. And more importantly, we've proven ourselves to be very efficient at spreading these pathogens through the extraordinary variety of transportation we use today.

Sars-2-CoV, the causative agent of COVID-19 – a soft, invisible creature – has shown itself to be tremendously powerful in disrupting the global socio-economic system as we know it. It has created a spiral of effects on human health, animal health, plant health and environmental health, which is destined to become transformative for us all. The challenge today is how to identify the obsolete pathways that must be abandoned and come up with new, undiscovered, alternative options. One way we can do this is by being open to ideas that come from other disciplines and by totally embracing a "thinking-out-of-the-box" approach. The tools and instruments we need to empower interdisciplinarity are abundant; the mindset is still in the pipeline. Here and now we have a unique opportunity to re-think health as a system and not as a series of private gardens.

But before you reinvent the wheel you should look at the wheels that were built before your time to understand how the concepts and knowledge evolved. Please join me, as we sit upon a star, looking at how the concept of health began, developed and matured over the centuries.

Let's share a journey as we see how systems were challenged with varying combinations of strength, formidable intuition and sheer luck.

Let's learn how many ideas and theories were discredited and attacked by the establishment, and how many scientists were shamed and persecuted.

Let's look together at what has driven change and explore how to enact a new way forward – now that COVID-19 has pointed us in the direction which nature intended.

We are the responsible players in the circle of life, and above all, guardians of the planet and defenders of its health.

It is a complex system.

To assist in this journey full of wonders and surprises, Daniele Mont D'Arpizio joined the project, playing the role of journalist and interviewer, asking the questions which would allow me to develop my argument, while Sara Agnelli, an adjunct professor with a PhD in Classics who works with me at the One Health Center of Excellence at the University of Florida, and Alberto Fioretti, an enthusiastic young man with a degree in philosophy, assisted with retrieving the documentation.

−6   A Maddening Idea

Ilaria, what is it that drives you to spark this wide-ranging debate about "Health" in the broadest sense of the word?

There's a desperate need for this conversation as we are fast approaching several tipping points. The extraordinary results we have obtained advancing the health of human beings are clear for all to see. But that doesn't mean that we should become complacent and rest on our laurels: there is definitely room for improvement on many fronts.

But before we get to discussing those areas of improvement, we need to be both vigilant and proactive in defending the inherent values of science. We know that science continually moves forward, the latest breakthrough leapfrogging over the one that came before, showing that what was true yesterday may not be true today and may be completely contradicted tomorrow. A typical example of this is the question of the least invasive technique to perform knee surgery – arthroscopy or open surgery? The answer is of course arthroscopy, but not if you asked this question prior to the 1970s. The advancement of science itself requires new ideas to upgrade existing dogmas. Good science is one step beyond.

But hasn't this always been the case? Why is it so important now?

Because it's time we put things into a new perspective and – why not – rethink our concept of "Health."

I still don't get it, so let's start with the basics. What defines "Health"?

Health has one inherent, paradoxical characteristic: you tend to think about it when it's not there; you appreciate it most when it's gone. This should already make us realize that, like other fundamental concepts such as beauty and justice, there's no single universal definition of health. So is health merely the absence of illness? And does "being healthy" necessarily refer to the entire organism or just the individual parts? Is health a state of mind and body or does it extend to the soul, whatever that word might mean to each of us? It is important to explain that overall, Health relates to different organisms and systems, it would be simplistic and misleading to place limitations on such a multifaceted concept.

But we still need to start from somewhere to frame the concept of Health. So, should we instead start by defining "illness"?

Well, of course it's easier to talk about illness than health. Illness is an additional element or condition, something you're experiencing. It's personal. In some ways, health lies in the shadow of illness, and as we've said often it's when you're ill that you realize what it means to be healthy. Humans began to think and conceptualize, and in order to understand the conditions of "health" and "disease," Greek medicine turned to the study of Nature (φύσις, *physis*), encompassing the totality of what exists, what is born, lives and dies. The so-called "Circle of life" that provides the landscape where the adventures of *The Lion King* play out.

This comprehensive, even holistic, approach developed back in ancient Greece was destined to realize its full potential in the modern era. The cornerstone of the rationale is as logical as it is obvious. And so many individuals have come to the same conclusion over the centuries, despite lacking all the necessary tools. Here's the bottom line: as human beings (*Homo sapiens*), we are totally dependent on other forms of life on Earth. So logically, it's in our best interest to protect, preserve and expand Health as a highly interdependent, multi-stakeholder resource that is an essential component of the overall ecosystem. Often, we make the mistake of thinking of Health as an asset and a resource that belongs to human beings alone, and only minimally concerns other living species. We now know that it just does not and cannot work like that.

Can you expand a little more?

Let's take it from a different angle. In the past, individuals were considered physically healthy when they didn't show any signs of disease, but our perspective today is far more articulated. For instance, the Constitution of the World Health Organization, signed in New York on July 22, 1946, opens with this statement: "Health is a state of complete physical, mental and social well-being and not merely the absence of disease or infirmity." This current and internationally recognized definition does not treat Health like a concept in a vacuum, as the mere absence of disease, but as a positive state of psycho-physical and even social well-being.

So why isn't this enough?

Because the time has come to update this definition, and make it even more inclusive. Just think back to a few decades ago, when there was a tendency to exclude mental health from the realm of physical health. Nowadays, it is universally accepted that your mental state can impact your physical Health. Today it seems obvious, but getting there was no small undertaking. In the same way, we know that social relationships play a fundamental role in maintaining health. Exercise can help against depression: a walk in the fresh air and sunshine is good for the mind. We now need to take the next big step forward by identifying new drivers, internal and external to the body, which can influence the health and well-being of an individual.

External drivers?

Exactly. The drivers that pertain to how our lives intersect with other lives, and how we all interact with the environment. Every one of us is connected to other animals (through the milk, eggs, honey and meat we consume, but also through the cat or the turtle that shares our home) to plants (bread, vegetables and fruit, beer and wine, the wood for our furniture) through to the inanimate world (water, air, sand, stone). Traditionally we see the environment as something external to our bodies, when we are in fact immersed in it. The environment is part of us, and thanks to food and water it builds our cells and sustains our lives and minds.

As an extreme comparison, humans are essentially sophisticated sponges absorbing the natural and unnatural components of our diet, of the environment, and necessary or unnecessary medical treatment. We are part of this greater system, that's for sure, but we also have an incredibly developed brain which has the capacity to influence our destiny, along with the destinies of our environment and of future generations.

Consider wheat, rice, and corn. Think of poultry and pork factories. Or the intentional introduction of the myxomatosis virus to cruelly control the Australian rabbit population. Or the historical widespread use of growth hormones in farm animals. And what about pandas? Or the northern white rhinos, whose numbers have dwindled to single digits?

And now we come to the big question.

In improving human health through overall social governance, have we done the best we can to preserve the environment and its resources? The crux of the question is this: can our species (since it looks like we're in charge) implement a new type of responsible innovation in health that is respectful of all stakeholders and sustainable at the same time? While this would be a big stretch for a creature with the mental capacity of an earthworm: *Homo sapiens* has the capability to make this happen.

That explains it. That's why after having trained and worked primarily as a virologist, today you're pursuing this new concept of One Health.

Actually, what I'm proposing is expanding the concept of One Health to help people rediscover the essence of the Circularity of Health.

But first we need to step back, and look at the origins of our concept of health. It's a different way to tackle current health challenges. And it gives us the chance to rethink all those concepts that have come up over and over so many times that they suddenly seem obvious, even if they aren't obvious at all.

I have to confess that history never really interested me as a student. I feel a bit guilty about that, but I really couldn't handle the slow pace of the subject. (Full disclosure, I found it incredibly boring!) But the time comes in your life when you see things from a different angle. And so after many years of super-focused scientific research, I felt the need to go back and take a closer look at those very historical areas I had previously neglected: history and philosophy, starting with the ancient world before Christ.

So, let's rewind…

And learn about the people and stories that proved the disruptive power of interdisciplinarity. I am revisiting the current concept of health, in keeping with some intuitions of the past, which we have mostly forgotten.

–5   Nothing to Begin With

Let's talk about the concept of health and healing in the pre-scientific era. Where should we start?

Pain hurts. And we humans have spent centuries trying to figure out what would help us deal with pain and illness. It's one of our most basic instincts, just like searching for food or seeking a safe place to sleep at night. All our efforts are really just attempts to slow down the unrelenting advance of death. Every day that you're alive is a day that brings you closer to death, so you might as well live life to its maximum potential feeling as good as you can. This explains why healers, barber-surgeons, medicine-men and women existed in practically all cultures. But since we're limiting our discussion to the Western world, and we need to start somewhere, we should begin with the ancient Greeks.

So, we're talking about 2,500 B.C.E. How did medical science develop in those days?

Long ago, there was still a lot to understand, and very few tools to work with to facilitate that understanding. However, one powerful resource proved to have the greatest impact on early explorations into health: the human brain. Its unique capabilities allowed early scholars to develop a multi-disciplinary convergence around the concept of health. Medicine, just like other sciences, emerged from philosophy, which at first was primarily focused on nature. Initially, ancient Greek medicine was framed by the more general cultural, philosophical and scientific context of the period, viewing human beings in all their innate complexity whilst taking into account environmental, biological and social dimensions. A sort of prehistoric One Health if you will.

The reasoning was that all organisms, animal and human, were composed of a combination of elements found in the cosmos. With this in mind, it was logical to deduce that good health was the result of the striking of a balance between these primary elements, whilst an imbalance would bring on illness. Taking certain preventative measures could avert an imbalance, and using certain therapies could help regain balance, with the environment playing a huge part in all this. The ancient Greeks embraced a broad approach to health and medicine, laying down a conceptual framework which still makes sense today.

How did the concept of health develop?

Understanding health hinges on physiology. The true definition of health can only be determined following the discovery of the functional mechanisms embedded in humans, animals, and plants. "How does it work?" was the question at the core of ancient medical thought.

So it follows that the notions of health (ὑγιεία, *hygiea*) and disease (νόσος, *nosos*) were built on the physiology of humors. This line of reasoning began with the writings of Alcmaeon (VI century B.C.E.), which were later organized in the works attributed to Hippocrates, (V–IV centuries B.C.E.), and subsequently enriched with the concept of *pneuma* by Aristotle (384/383–322 B.C.E.).[1] Finally, it would fall to Galen (circa 130–200 C.E.) to take further the work of his predecessors, condense it and make sense of over 700 years' worth of their theories, attempting to redefine the whole human being as "one coherent system." Seven hundred years to work it all out... to the next level.

In those days, scientists had very limited factual knowledge to work with: they had to draw an imaginary framework for the concept of health, but they had no evidence, no data, no parameters at their disposal. They didn't know how extensive the framework was supposed to be, so they didn't have the slightest idea how to work within that framework. At the time they knew nothing of cells or microbes; nobody had lightbulbs, microscopes or cameras available to illuminate or immortalize such detail. They could only work on what they could see with the naked eye. The rest came from the power of the mind.

Returning to the humors, was this theory really so important?

There is no doubt that it was a fundamental starting point. The ancient Greeks hypothesized humors in connection with the theory of the four elements (earth, air, water, and fire), which formed the basis of the medicine and physiology of the day. Hippocrates (generally considered the founder of medicine) tells us that it was his son-in-law Polybus (V-IV centuries B.C.E.), also a physician, who linked the four fundamental elements to the humors, that is, the four different fluids which circulate inside the body. These fluids (blood, yellow bile, black bile and phlegm) were in turn associated with the properties hot/cold and dry/wet, respectively. This became the dominant theory of the time and persisted until quite recently. "Learn how it works" was largely a question of using the imagination, since human dissection was not allowed. In other scientific disciplines such as chemistry and physics, knowledge was also still at a very early stage of development.

What was the point of this theory?

It was an attempt to explain the pathophysiology of the human body – how it works and how we get sick – based on the assumption that our bodily fluids are in a constant state of flux. This dynamic was believed to be affected by changes in the seasons, in diet and in behavior. According to Aristotle, the fundamental elements went through reciprocal transformations contingent on the hot/cold and dry/wet states: just like earth, air, fire, and water, so did the basic ingredients of living organisms. Finally, extrapolating from Aristotelian tradition, Galen developed the theory of the mixture of humors as the unique characteristic that constitutes the human body. As we transition from childhood to adulthood and then to old age, this internal equilibrium is subject to change. So, the key to living a healthy life was keeping the humors in the proper balance with the help of a physician. This concept facilitated a major step forward in active health management.

So according to this perspective, what is health? And how can we overcome illness and regain health again?

In general terms, according to humoralism, health was directly affected by too much or too little of any one of the four bodily fluids. The term *eucrasia* (in Greek εὐκρασία, "good mixture") indicated a proper and harmonious balance of the body's humoral elements, which was the key to good health. The opposite was an imbalance or *discrasia* (in Greek δυσκρασία, "bad mixture") between the bodily fluids, which would lead to illness. Too much of one element takes away from the others. So without any other fixed parameters, health and illness were all about balance and imbalance.

In practical terms, how did this translate into therapies?

Objective, scientific data were non-existent in those days, and it was particularly complicated to move from theory to practice. People did their best with what was available at the time in terms of knowledge, instruments and means of intervention. Attempts to rebalance the humors included blood-letting and purges, together with a proper diet and a good relationship with the environment. Humors were seen as being dependent on nutrition, breathing and quality of life, all tying into the relationship between the human body and nature, time and history. This emerging concept of health included – for the first time – the space inside and outside the body.

Do the politics of the time influence health?

Yes – a lot. One of the most famous principles of Hippocratic medicine says that democracy produces healthy citizens, while tyranny generates ill subjects.

So you're saying that the ancient Greek idea of health was already more inclusive than our own?

That's right. Their focus on the human body was never disconnected from the environmental, physical, and social context. Once upon a time it didn't make sense for physicians to reason in terms of health and disease as being removed from the outside world: different climatic configurations (or "constitutions") led to the different body shapes and traits that characterized different populations. The color of the skin, the shape of the eyes and the nose were all influenced by the environment. This made sense then and makes even more sense now after Darwin.

According to Galen, the balance between the humors shaped the temperament of the organs and of the overall organism, and all this in turn was affected by environmental and behavioral factors. The changing seasons, and in particular the prevailing environmental conditions, had a specific influence on the delicate balance between health and illness. This allowed physicians to predict various types of diseases and how they would evolve. Primary causes of illness were believed to be heat, cold, humidity. In a treatise entitled *On Airs, Waters, and Places*, Hippocrates advised travelling physicians to "consider the seasons of the year, and what effects each of them produces." He went on to expound upon the health implications of "the winds, the heat and the cold," "the qualities of the waters," rain and drought, each city's unique position in the surrounding landscape, and even whether its inhabitants were given to excess and passivity or discipline and courage. "These things one ought to consider most attentively," he wrote. So the concept of climate's profound influence on health is nothing new.

Theories from a thousand years ago are teaching us something today?

One lesson we can learn from that time is that we should always be aware of the link between the human body and the socio-physical environment. Also, many texts from the *Corpus Hippocraticum* and Galen's work focused on prevention, which included a healthy diet, exercise, rest, and sex. So, the doctor-philosopher is someone who takes care of the patient in relation to his or her living space and lifestyle. As a matter of fact, medical and pharmaceutical metaphors were often used in classical times to describe the role of philosophy. An early example is from Democritus, who drew a parallel between the role of wisdom as a medicine in treating the soul: "Medicine heals bodily illness, while wisdom frees the soul from suffering."

That sounds very modern…

The theory of humors influenced the concept of health as it was developing up until the sixteenth century at least. And even after that, the ideas of Hippocrates and Galen continued to carry weight as recently as the mid-nineteenth century. This is because, considering the limitations in knowledge and technology of the times, the theory was surprisingly insightful. The underlying logic made it possible to formulate explanatory hypotheses even when phenomena clashed with pre-existing ideas.

Does this mean we have to go back to leeches and bloodletting?

Of course not! Not at all. Although in a pre-scientific society these procedures, if properly managed, probably provided some relief. That may well have been mostly due to what we now recognize as the placebo effect. In any case, the theory of humors was conceptually sound and offered rich insights, even for today's world.

Recognizing the link between mental and physical health has come about extremely late in our history, and in some respects, this link is still widely ignored, even ridiculed. Humoral medicine acknowledges the existence of a highly complex level of interconnections within the body, and between the body and mind. It extends beyond the individual, encompassing a variety of external factors. It implies a dependence on nature.

Although the theory is fundamentally flawed and inadequate, the logic and wisdom in its rules and mechanisms is still palpable. This is immensely relevant today because, unlike in the past, we do have the tools to understand, measure and study interconnections which were unthinkable even fifty years ago. Just think of the relationship between climate change and the incidence of allergies, or the spread of mosquito-borne diseases. The time has come for the medical community to reclaim that intuition and those ancient ideas of complexity – because today we have the tools we need and the right mindset to understand the ramifications of these multiple interconnections. Hopefully, this new three-dimensional understanding can guide us along our path to improving wellbeing in a sustainable way.

Notes

[1] The post-classical Latin term *pneuma* is borrowed from the ancient Greek noun πνεῦμα, which means "wind," "breath," and from the verb πνέω, "to blow," "to breathe." In ancient physiology, *pneuma* was used to describe an air- or spirit-like material, derived from inhaled air, which travelled through the arteries either alone or in combination with blood, and circulated throughout the body. In Hellenistic Greek the term also indicated "spirit," and more specifically the vital, conscious component in every living organism – corresponding in meaning to the Latin noun *spiritus*.

−4 Art Becomes a Tool for Science

So, Ilaria, according to the theory of humors, health and well-being of humans, animals, plants, and the environment were all inter-connected. What can we do today to empower this vision and regain that sense of inclusivity?

Well, first we need to explore a few other drivers and take a leap forward in time to the Middle Ages.

The Middle Ages? What does that have to do with science and health?

Quite a lot, really. When we think of the Middle Ages, we immediately picture burning witches (something which regrettably really happened, but mostly later, in the seventeenth century). It's considered a period of violence and barbarity, often even directed against science, but that isn't the whole story. If we look at how things developed over time, we'll get a different picture: we'll see that periods of apparent stagnation were followed by flashes of brilliant innovation.

How did people think about health in the Middle Ages?

The general consensus is that at that time there was some confusion as to what was and wasn't science.

Remember, this was before Galileo and his contemporaries came on the scene, so their ideas weren't around to influence the way society thought. Science at the time did not involve any formal scientific method and was not yet evidence-based. It was something more like magic, left to the whims of supreme beings and supernatural forces.

In fact, health was still referred to as *salus* – essentially centering on the salvation of the soul. There was a sort of rivalry between the health of the body versus the soul, with the latter clearly prevailing. At times heresy (the illness of the soul) struck more fear in the hearts of people than the plague. And let's not forget, conventional wisdom at the time held that the main cause of disease was the wrath of God, sent down to punish sinners who had lost their way.

That doesn't sound like fertile ground for advances in medicine...

Yet there were advances, and important ones too. But to recognize them, we need to look beyond the borders of Europe. I'm referring to what we now call the Middle East, a place which in our collective imagination is often associated with war and terrorism today. But back then it was the epicenter of ground-breaking accomplishments in medical science. In fact, there and then – in the Middle East in the Middle Ages – the theory of medicine was preserved, cultivated and perpetuated, surmounting enormous linguistic, cultural and religious barriers. And all the while Western Europe languished.

What drove the process of medical progress in the Middle East?

We can think of it as the result of a process of inclusive thinking and creative reinterpretation, expanding and enriching Greco-Roman philosophy and science thanks to contributions from other cultures we haven't mentioned yet, particularly Islam. In fact, it was the exposure to other cultures, along with widespread translation and reinterpretation, which helped shore up the foundations of medicine and health.

This was little short of a miracle, considering all the barriers that had to be to overcome: linguistic, logistic, and cultural, to name but a few. So just think, in Medieval times Syriac scholars acted as liaisons between the Byzantine Empire and Islam, and through their initial translation and reinterpretation, the great Greek authors travelled from the Mediterranean to the Arab world. Clearly the lines of communication couldn't rely on high speed internet… instead spreading information meant getting on a horse and riding for hundreds of kilometers. But despite the relative lack of speed in communications, this linguistic and cultural interconnection turned science into something different from what it used to be. Science didn't just borrow the framework from the Greek vision, but expanded on it.

For example, science introduced a new universal language: Arabic numerals. Did you know that what we call Arabic numerals today (the numbers 1 through 9) actually originated several centuries earlier in India? Anyway, try to imagine science without Arabic numerals. How could we write up our data the old way, with Roman numerals? Remember, the Romans used a much more complex system to express magnitude: $I = 1$, $III = 3$ but $IV = 4$ (effectively 5–1) and $VI = 6$ (effectively 5+1), $X = 10$ (introducing a new letter code). So overall the whole thing really was much more complicated. Imagine everyday objects like license plates without Arabic numerals – we would need XXXL-size plates! Very importantly, Arabic numerals introduced something new that Roman numerals had never contemplated: the concept of zero.

If Arabic numerals became so popular, there must have been a reason why. They likely facilitated how scientists summarized data, enabling them to communicate with one another more easily. And who knows, maybe without Arabic numerals, the scientific revolution wouldn't have even been possible. Here again, circularity and interconnections come into play. Loaded with "exogenous pollen" as the means for natural dissemination of innovation, Greco-Roman culture reappeared in the West, mainly via Spain, enriched by the observations of the great Muslim doctors and scientists and encoded with Arabic numerals. Scientists like pollinators carry pollen as the insects do, between disciplines and theories.

Cross-fertilization? What does pollination have to do with innovation?

Pollination is simply a metaphor to show that interconnection is fundamental! Pollinators carry pollen as they fly from flower to flower and fertilize the females. It is a way to transform "kinetic energy" (energy that an object possesses due to its motion) to enable development and progress. Knowledge is a big, big word, I agree, but I think it fits here – knowledge itself can be described as an infinite number of interconnected communicating vessels. Dynamic, not static. Liquid – or rather circular if I may.

In the Middle Ages, Islamic culture led the way for the simple reason that it was wide open to external influence. This culture knew how to absorb knowledge, and then reformulate and adapt it. The Arab conquerors recognized and appreciated the value of Greek philosophy and Indian mathematics. (That actually seems like quite a challenge – human narcissism would lead any conqueror to automatically down-play any areas of excellence of the conquered.)

And while Islamic culture was gradually processing and assimilating these innovative ideas, it crossed paths with the Persian civilization and human knowledge took a quantum leap forward. For centuries Persia had represented a beacon for science and culture, especially medicine, attracting the brightest Arab students who would go to study at Persian universities. An illustrious example is the first Arab doctor we know of (Al-Harith ibn Kalada (d. 634/635), Muhammad's personal physician) who studied in Gondeshapur, Persia.[1]

How did these exchanges, or cross-fertilizations as you call them, come about?

Just like they do in nature. You asked me about pollen and cross-fertilization; well, the process resembles what happens with bees when they move around and carry pollen which fertilizes the egg cells of flowers. Bees are unaware of their role as fertilizers, and they're definitely NL. (You may be wondering what that means... keep reading!) One thing that utterly amazes me about this period is how far afield intellectuals used to move around, just like bees. And they did so in spite of the dangers and the lack of infrastructure. It was normal to travel for days back then, often on foot or on horseback, to reach a particular school and to study there, or to seek out exceptional teachers to learn from, and then bring this new knowledge back home. And all whilst contending with immense barriers: language, culture and, of course, religion.

Today it's a different story: with one click you can travel to the past, present or future. And if you don't understand the language there's always Google Translate, which is certainly a great start, compared to the years of study it used to take. In those days, the first universities were being established, and the *clerici vagantes*[2] were embarking on their explorative journeys. These were the first itinerant scholars or "fellows," whilst the House of Wisdom in what would become Baghdad was the hub for what was truly a system of "brain circulation." In other words, it was already clear even then that scholars have to move, because only by exchanging ideas and experiences can knowledge expand.

But there you've really lost me. So you're saying the Dark Ages really weren't dark, Islam isn't a fundamentally obscurantist culture, and "brain circulation" isn't a recent phenomenon.

Here, we touch on the high points of a great success story, and we really need to acknowledge the positive aspects that are often overlooked. So, for instance, if we have gene therapies today, it's thanks to the overall expansion and maturation of our scientific knowledge. From this perspective, we could say that the Middle Ages were a time of transformation for medicine and the concept of health in a myriad of ways. During this period specialized knowledge was being developed, but at the same time physician-scientist-scholars were still focused on their holistic vision of humankind and our place in the universe. There was also a growing realization that scholars had to move towards centers of excellence, to facilitate the generation of new theories of health management. That realization is even more evident today.

… and so we fast forward to the Renaissance.

That's right, it was the beginning of a colossal convergence of knowledge which shook the very foundations of Classical thought. A new vision, a tapestry weaving together science, technology and art – all embodied in the genius of Leonardo da Vinci, the prototypical Renaissance man. But he wasn't the only one. There are other unsung heroes who are no less consequential in the history of medicine, such as Girolamo Fracastoro (circa 1476–1553). He was considered one of the most brilliant doctors of all time, together with Andreas Vesalius (1514–1564), the founder of modern anatomy.

Why was anatomy so important?

It was fundamental, because it made the transition possible from a traditional concept of medicine belonging to the sphere of the arts, to medicine as a true science. Medicine was considered in medieval universities as an *ars*, a subject which in some ways was overshadowed by philosophy or theology. Science came into the picture through novel, previously unthinkable approaches based on direct observation of the human body (primarily through the dissection of corpses). Without this, there would have been no scientific grounding for a number of other disciplines ranging from physiology to surgery to neuroscience.

You mentioned Andreas Vesalius. Why was his work so influential?

He was a game changer. The field of anatomy is divided into a before and after *Fabrica*, his magnum opus. Scientific rigor and artistic talent converged in Vesalius, and thanks to the astounding anatomic drawings accompanying his works, generations of doctors were trained using a revolutionary method, because he drew his illustrations using perspective. If we look a modern anatomy atlas today, little has changed since Vesalius' inspired work. By uniting art and science, he made science emerge as something tangible, something real. Art became a means of communicating science.

But who was Vesalius?

He was born in Brussels, the son of the apothecary to the Imperial Court, and became one of the greatest doctors of his time. The Emperor's personal physician, in fact. Supposedly Charles V and his son Philip II wouldn't even go for a walk without him by their side.

From an early age Vesalius had one mission: the study of anatomy. This is why, as a young student in Paris, he began visiting cemeteries and the gallows to gather "research material." And this is what prompted him to move to Padua, in Italy, drawn by the intellectual freedom there – and by the availability of corpses to dissect.

As a great example of "brains on the move," Vesalius left Flanders and at 23 graduated as a Doctor of Medicine at the University of Padua. He was immediately nominated professor of surgery, with the proviso that he would teach anatomy, which he did in his own unique way. During his lessons he used a complete human skeleton and individual bones, and relied on his drawings to illustrate how blood vessels and nerves threaded their way through this structural support. But eventually his meticulous studies led him to realize that what he was teaching his students was inaccurate. Why? Because at that time, anatomy was still essentially based on Galen's works. But this didn't quite correspond to what Vesalius could see with his own eyes each time he examined a corpse.

So, what was wrong?

As he continued with his observations, he realized that there were mistakes in Galenic anatomy: for instance, the structures of both the upper and lower jaw looked different; the liver, which according to Galen had five lobes, actually only had four. After pouring over the ancient texts, he concluded that Galen's human anatomy was based on dissecting animals, in particular monkeys. The number of differences lead Vesalius to realize there was an urgent need to revise this entire body of knowledge, and that this revised knowledge had to be made public and easily accessible.

And is that why his works were so revolutionary?

De humani corporis fabrica (or *Fabrica*), published in 1543, was immediately perceived as a new dawn breaking in anatomical science, thanks to its sweeping scope, its rigorous accuracy and the inherent beauty and depth of more than 300 illustrations. With this treatise Vesalius redefined the subject and openly defied Galen's authority by correcting his assumptions and errors. Ultimately, Vesalius found the courage to challenge two thousand years of knowledge. And how did he do it? Through art.

Of all the many remarkable pieces of his work, his exquisite woodblocks are what we most often think of.

Yes, so true! The *Fabrica* wasn't just a milestone in the history of medicine, it was also an artistic masterpiece stunningly illustrated with the drawings of Jan Steven van Calcar (1499–1546), a fellow countryman of Vesalius and a pupil of Titian, and skillfully published by Johannes Herbst of Basel (known as *Oporinus*, 1507–1568). The topics were presented in the order of Vesalius' teaching syllabus: bones, muscles, blood vessels and nerves, internal organs and the brain. Leafing through the pages, your eye is immediately caught by the illustrations, which are some of the most sophisticated anatomical representations ever made.

But these amazing illustrations were not just an aesthetic choice. Vesalius wanted to drive home his central point: anatomy was essential to medicine, and the only way to advance the study of anatomy was through direct observation.

I'd like to focus on one operational issue for just a moment. (For the squeamish among you, you're better off skipping right to the next question.) Studying anatomy is a dirty job – from direct observation to completely dissecting corpses under surgical conditions, while taking notes. When you perform a task that spans from life into death, it forces you come face to face with death and one of its inevitable effects: decomposition. And remember, in those days there were no gloves, no masks or sharp scalpels, and of course no refrigerators; the job of dissecting was unbelievably crude, disgusting even. But through his example Vesalius showed that the only path forward to acquiring new knowledge must rely on studying human biological material, as opposed to mindlessly repeating outdated teachings. It was a revolution in every sense of the word: the birth of medicine as science.

How did his contemporaries react to this?

Some took it very badly. The traditionalists never forgave him. What's more, his own teacher in Paris, Jacques Dubois (known as Jacobus Sylvius, 1478–1555), a fervent Galenist, even went so far as to call him insane, describing him as "monstrous" and "the most dangerous example of ignorance, ingratitude, arrogance and godlessness." Even Gabriele Falloppio (1523–1562), who took Vesalius's teaching post in Padua, condemned him, though with less caustic words. Vesalius was insulted, reviled, mocked. Isn't that the way it always goes? If you decide to stand against the tide, you must be prepared to pay a heavy personal price for defending your ideas.

How did Vesalius react?

He left his position in Padua, burnt all his notes, and moved to Spain to become the king's personal physician. For the rest of his life he continued to defend his discoveries against criticism by some of his contemporaries, but by the time he turned 28 the most productive period of his life was over. He died on the island of Zante in the Ionian Sea in 1564, not yet fifty years old, returning from one of his journeys. What happened? Well, according to one version of the story, he had travelled to the Holy Land, either on a pilgrimage or as some sort of penance, allegedly after being accused of dissecting living bodies. What we know for sure is that he never made it back. Perhaps he would have liked to return to Venice or Padua, and defend his work again and – why not? – maybe even go back to teaching at the university. But the hardships of the journey, and possibly a plague epidemic, would in the end prove fatal. Think of how ironic life – or rather death – can be. Vesalius was the man who had drawn bodies that were studied by doctors the world over – yet his own body was never found.

Why is Vesalius still so relevant today?

In Vesalius I clearly see an example of someone inspired by what I believe was a mission: a man who created something extraordinary, not only in its content but also its form, the way he presented it. One of the great revolutions in Vesalius' work is its artistic quality, achieved through the skillful use of images of dissected corpses. The drawings are superb, and thanks to the use of perspective, they achieve an unprecedented degree of realism. For the first time, optical enhancements were used expertly to enable students to come to a deeper understanding of the complexities of human anatomy. Perspective techniques gave students new 3D imaging of the human body. That was and remains quite an achievement.

Here's something else that's interesting to think about. Would we see so many US Study Abroad programs, or European Erasmus exchange programs, if it weren't for the "proto-Europeans" – first and foremost, Vesalius?

A real artistic treasure.

Leafing through the *Fabrica*, even electronically (go take a look, it's just a click away), you'll find even the legends striking. Vesalius identifies certain parts of each drawing and provides relevant notes, using a style which he may have copied from books on botany. With this method, he introduces a level of clarity that had never been seen before. To say nothing of the perfect harmony between innovative content, artistic sensibility and graphic technique, developed by Vesalius in an attempt to give students a front row seat to observe his dissections. It is a masterpiece which still inspires awe today, notwithstanding the conditions the author worked under to finish it, without any means of preserving corpses or protecting them from decay.

You mentioned that Vesalius was a sort of Copernicus of medicine...

By extraordinary coincidence (or was it?), the two luminaries published their master works almost simultaneously (June 1543). First was *De revolutionibus orbium coelestium*, the book in which Nicolaus Copernicus presented the details of the heliocentric system first suggesting that the Earth orbited around a stationary Sun; and then just a few weeks later came Vesalius' *De humani corporis fabrica*. Now, it's unlikely that the two ever met, yet it's still extraordinary that both, each one a major scientist of this period, travelled to Italy to study. Proof positive that there was a time when Italy was the center of a vast network of interconnections which crisscrossed the whole of Europe. Padua especially, where both Vesalius and Copernicus studied and where William Harvey also graduated. (A few decades later Harvey would describe the cardiovascular system – another fundamental discovery for the birth of the new branch of medical science.) So it comes as no surprise that the science historian Herbert Butterfield called Padua "the birthplace of the scientific revolution."

And so, we come to modern science.

Modern scientific thought began to emerge in Western history during the Renaissance, even though substantial progress was made in the seventeenth century. We're talking about the attentive observations of reality (something which Aristotle did as well), substantiated by repeated experiments, the innovative use of mathematics, and trial and error (the Galilean method). A new model of understanding was born, verifiable by anybody (at least in theory) and based more on facts than on tradition or intuition.

In hindsight, so-called "ancient science" was actually rather basic, an assortment of notions often with blurred borders between very different fields and very little in common. In all fairness, it's true that the "founding fathers of science" had to start somewhere, and without a robust conceptual framework many ideas were difficult to grasp enough on their own.

The theory of humors gave us a holistic vision which blamed illness mainly on imbalances between these four body substances. The assumption was that too much or too little of the same humors directly influenced health and temperament. It still seems plausible today: you get mad when you're stuck in a traffic jam and you end up with a headache. But change came, and with it the scientific revolution bearing the foundations for the modern world. Citizens and scientists today are all indebted to Galileo and to other pioneers who at some point decided to bring about a change. With a capital C.

One aspect you keep going back to is interconnections.

The tale we're telling is all about interconnections: between cultures, languages and countries, but also between art and science. Science is not always rigidly divided into sectors, quite the opposite. The most successful scientists often borrow innovative ideas, methods, and perspectives from different fields. These stories help us understand that even in the past, scientists' horizons weren't limited to a single country: interdisciplinarity and "brain circulation" have always existed. This is one more reason we should support scientific migrants today.

We're talking about a transition which evolved over several centuries. Why did it take so long to overcome the old system?

Because the groundwork had to be laid for a different future. If, for example, we look at the scientific revolution, we should remember that it wasn't an instantaneous breakthrough: it would take centuries to overcome certain entrenched notions and superstitions. The story goes that for years Galileo himself continued to write horoscopes for a fee to supplement his lecturer's salary. New methodologies to advance scientific knowledge forced scholars to become increasingly specialized. This marked the beginning of a so-called "vertical approach" which led to a detailed improvement in overall scientific understanding. But it came at the cost of that broad outlook which had characterized scholarly activity in the past, and reciprocal "pollination" between different disciplines and cultures was lost. This is why it's essential to remember and revisit figures such as Leonardo da Vinci (1452–1519) and Vesalius. And by the way, da Vinci, whose death five hundred years ago was commemorated in 2019, was very probably also NL.

The contrast with the speed of movement today is startling. In the past the logical thread of an illuminating or revolutionary idea was often hidden behind a veil of uncertainty. Today we know much more and can access it all with a click. Do you want to find out about the anatomy of the platypus, that duck-billed egg-laying beaver-like animal that only lives in Oceania? Just type and click.

This means that finding innovative solutions should be simpler. We can assume that the information we need to make a huge discovery or invention is already out there, just waiting for us to find it. So, what lies between data and a huge discovery? Fundamentally, an idea. And ideas are much easier to come by if you go looking for them beyond your immediate mental boundaries, and with an open mind. Developing and optimizing investigative mechanisms is easier today than ever before.

Notes

[1] Gondeshapur was a Persian city in the south-western region of what is today the province of Khuzestan in Iran. For centuries, the city was the intellectual heart of the Sassanid Empire (224–651) and housed the famed "Academy of Gondeshapur." During the sixth and seventh centuries the Academy became the foremost medical center from East to West.

[2] *Clerici vagantes*, "wandering clerics," is a medieval Latin term, describing students who travelled throughout Europe to take lessons the four most important academic subjects in the Middle Ages (Philosophy, Medicine, Law, Theology). These faculties were often offered at different European universities located all over the continent. This experience was known as *peregrinatio academica*, a complex interplay of individual interests, organizational conditions at the study location, and not least political factors.

−3 Never From Within, Always From Beyond

In the previous chapter you mentioned how Andrea Vesalius, who was considered the father of modern anatomy, probably died of the plague.

Yes, that's true. The Plague (specifically the bubonic plague caused by *Yersinia pestis*) was the most feared enemy of the time, the "relentlessly deadly" epidemic. Pestilence had been regarded for centuries as a form of divine punishment; it was associated with revenge and retribution both in the Iliad and in the Bible. It struck both rich and poor, never respecting class or position: it was a true social leveler. We must also bear in mind that until the early sixteenth century, "plague" was still a generic term used to describe virtually any disease. That certainly makes it more difficult to understand which specific illnesses were referred to as plague. History may well have underestimated the impact of this devastating disease in the pre-vaccine and pre-antibiotic era.

How were infectious diseases perceived?

With great fear and little understanding. Imagine being blindfolded and trying to walk a tightrope. Well, the scholars of that time really were blindfolded, given that they couldn't even begin to imagine the myriad of parallel worlds they were about to discover. Microorganisms still lived in a hidden realm. However, what was understood since ancient times was that certain diseases somehow moved from one person to another, in some cases spreading to geographical areas beyond the original outbreak. But for centuries no one could figure out how or why that happened. The classicists thought that epidemics were caused by natural events like the misalignment of the stars, volcanic eruptions, marshland vapors, filth and stenches emanating from putrid, decaying bodies. In short, no evidence-based theories.

An initial attempt at preventative medicine, and a logical first step, was to physically distance healthy people from sick ones who could be a source of disease transmission. To protect themselves, doctors started wearing masks shaped like elongated beaks – imagine what some Venetian masks look like and you'll get the idea. The beaks were filled with straw and aromatic essences that supposedly acted like filters. This was the inspiration behind the forerunners of modern HEPA filter masks. The long shape of the masks allowed doctors to keep a safe distance from their patients. The longer the beak, the further away – and the safer – the doctor was.

And what about plague-spreaders? The Italian writer Alessandro Manzoni wrote extensively about them in his descriptions of the dreaded 1630 plague of Milan.

Even medical experts like Alessandro Tadino (1580–1661), who fought tirelessly against the spread of the plague, believed in the existence of plague-spreaders. At some level that's understandable: even today, in the age of technology and information, conspiracy theories are everywhere. Ultimately having a culprit to blame is paradoxically reassuring (the plague-spreaders of the past, or today perhaps a doctor administering a vaccine). We feel better when we think it's somebody else's fault, and we're not forced to question our beliefs or behaviors. Most importantly, it absolves us of all responsibility.

Given how widespread the disease was, how could the "experts" of the time not notice the mechanisms of disease transmission right before their very eyes?

Here we come to a turning point in history. Observations suggested that classical medical theory, based on humors, could no longer provide satisfactory answers. Humoralism correctly emphasized the environment's influence on health, but was missing several essential pieces of the puzzle such as microorganisms, those pathogenic agents responsible for practically all infectious diseases.

Going back to the plague, Manzoni also made frequent mention of quarantine stations or lazarets. Were they really that dreadful?

The one described in Manzoni's book *The Betrothed* certainly sounds like a hellhole, with no water and thirty people to a room. They were forced to sleep on the floor or on rotten straw, eating bread made out of a foul mix of inedible ingredients. Environments like those were unhealthy per se, with or without the plague. But surprisingly in some cases these quarantine stations, with proper upkeep and under less extreme circumstances, actually contributed to limiting disease transmission; sometimes patients even got better.

Today one of the first steps for preventing the spread of disease is to isolate the people who are already infected. Quarantine – forty days of isolation imposed on ships in the fourteenth century when they arrived in port from plague-infested areas – is still in use. Forty days: that's how long Noah spent on the ark, or Moses on Mount Sinai; how long it took to perform the embalming process in Ancient Egypt, or for a woman to be purified after childbirth.

How did the lazarets come to be?

Italy was a great laboratory for understanding how infrastructures, and more generally the environment, could play a role in the spread of disease. Many aspects of disease were still unknown, but person-to-person contact was believed to favor transmission. People interacting with other people. And from here, the interconnection between human health and the environment which could either accelerate or even extinguish outbreaks.

To control this interconnection, guidelines and procedures were developed and put into practice on a multitude of islands serendipitously close at hand.

The city of Venice with its peculiar geographical layout was the perfect spot to test a rudimentary "epidemiological" approach for the first time. As a major trading hub, Venice saw a constant flow of merchants and travelers from all over the world. It soon became apparent that the risk of disease transmission and the spread of disease were closely tied to people's movements and to their contacts with locals. But bear in mind interpersonal contact in those days was quite different from what it is now, and certain parts of the lagoon city could remain separated from the rest rather easily. So isolating patients on selected islands within the Venetian lagoon was a solution that provided a simple natural barrier to the spread of disease.

Lazarets actually turned into laboratories that gave rise to new medical practices: experience translated into concepts and procedures which would later prove essential in controlling infectious diseases. For instance, it became clear that people could be contagious even if they didn't show any clinical symptoms. What's more, for the first time, people realized that infection could also be spread through personal items or inanimate objects – think of a single fountain in a park that everyone in the neighborhood drinks from.

The lazaret ecosystem provided evidence of how vital it was to avoid contact not only with the sick, but even with their personal effects and clothing, as well as corpses and the rooms where bodies had been laid. Most importantly the lazarets themselves began to implement additional control measures such as destroying everything which was suspected of being infected. A form of "proto-sanitization": it wasn't yet sterilization as we conceive it today, but at least it was a step in the right direction. Bit by bit, the age-long enigma of disease transmission began to unravel, with the caveat that it would take an exceptionally long time for it to be definitively understood.

Who was responsible for laying the groundwork for understanding infectious diseases in Venice at that time?

A new and audacious idea was published in 1546 by a contemporary of Vesalius, a man called Girolamo Fracastoro. He was a physician, philosopher, and astronomer. Today we would call him a disruptive innovator. He was arguably one of the most brilliant doctors of all time. His ground-breaking treatise published in Venice focused on the possible mechanics of disease transmission, *De contagione et contagiosis morbis et curatione* ("On Contagion and Contagious Diseases and Cure"). This may not look like a big deal for us today, but we have to remember that the essential tools for verifying his intuition wouldn't be invented for another three centuries.

In order to make a discovery you first need to imagine it and Fracastoro was gifted with boundless imagination. He was the first to hypothesize that infections were the result of disease-carrying microorganisms that could multiply inside the body and infect others via the breath or other forms of contact. So he provided a cause (microbes) with multiple consequences (illness and contagion). A leap forward in the right direction that was beyond the mental limitations of his peers.

Let's put the immensity of his thinking into perspective. In those days, the perceived range of existence was constrained by what could be observed with the naked eye. If we compare what was visible then to what is visible today – from distant stars thousands of light-years away, to corpuscles within the cells of living organisms, to the smallest molecules – we can say that Fracastoro lacked at least 99.9 per cent of the information he needed to understand the mechanisms of disease transmission. Yet he was able to imagine those very microbes which would only be discovered – and become visible – many years later.

How was such an extraordinary insight possible?

Fracastoro began by studying a widespread and greatly feared disease known as the "French Disease" or syphilis. Based on these studies, in 1530 in Verona he published the poem *Syphilis sive De morbo gallico* ("Of Syphilis, or of the French Disease"): a scientific treatise in Latin verse, another perfect example of "contamination" between science and the humanities. Starting from fieldwork and clinical observations, Fracastoro came to realize that some key factors conflicted with the old humoral doctrine, and required a new explanation. The time had come when it was no longer possible to simply augment the old doctrine, as new observations just wouldn't fit into that old theoretical framework. The drivers of infectious disease spread were obvious in many ways; entire family groups would fall ill, or networks of people who had been in contact with one another. These events could not be explained simply by stench and filth.

With his next treatise, *De contagione et contagiosis morbis*, Fracastoro would build a new paradigm, challenging the idea that unhealthy smells and odors – or miasma[1] – were the cause of illness. A bad smell can obviously make you queasy, but it certainly can't cause fever or pestilence, so there had to be something else that was causing a spreading sickness within the bad smell. Or more specifically, there had to be something else. This change in the perception of a problem is something that occurs in science in general and in the study of health in particular: truth is constantly evolving. A fact is only true at a particular time, before a new truth emerges in the face of new evidence. At some point you have to decide either to respond to what pulls you forward, or stick to what holds you back and what you've always been taught. And it's not an easy decision.

So, what did Fracastoro decide to do?

To move forward. His first great idea was to give miasma tangible form. He believed that it was neither the vapors given off by rot, nor the "corrupt" air, but rather a poison – *virus* in Latin[2] – which he now considered the real agent of epidemic diseases. And so the enemy began to take a physical state: it suddenly existed, and so it could be fought and defeated.

A huge leap forward.

Yes, and that was only the beginning. Fracastoro also understood that whatever was contained within miasma, it could spread and multiply. In other words, it could move from an infected body to a healthy one, sickening the new healthy host. The newly contaminated individual would then amplify the spread of the disease to other healthy individuals, making them sick too. So through his reasoning on disease transmission, Fracastoro not only imagined pathogens – he was able to define them. He believed the "material" component of miasma to be *seminaria*, small seeds of infection which could flourish in the right environment. Just like seeds in the ground, the *seminaria contagiorum* were small, invisible disease-transmitting bodies, which could grow and flourish in the fertile "terrain" of favorable body humors. A good compromise between the old dogmatic humoral theory and the intuition of an animated microcosm.

How did these "seeds" spread?

According to Fracastoro, epidemic diseases primarily afflicted the poor, and of course filth and malnutrition didn't help. It was quite an astute observation at the time, and is still very true today. Fracastoro believed that *seminaria* favored the *crudissimi* (raw) humors typical of the *pauperes* (poor). Remember that the poor often lived in overcrowded environments, crammed into shacks and shanties, hospices, and taverns. They were soldiers, pilgrims, beggars, and homeless wanderers. Clearly local gatherings facilitated the spread of disease, but there is something else that brings people into contact, facilitating this interaction: movement.

Proximity is a critical factor in our discussion. Why? Because disease transmission occurs between an infected organism and a susceptible one, and in the vast majority of cases, it implies physical proximity. Through infection, people could amplify and spread disease: the *seminaria* would release themselves from the surface of the body, like leaves falling during a windy autumn day. When you introduce the concept of "proximity," you have the explanation for the dissemination of disease. That was Fracastoro's great intuition: it was the *seminaria*, not rotten or putrid air, which spread infectious disease.

What was Fracastoro's contribution to the understanding of epidemic diseases?

What he did was reformulate, rethink, and reinvent ancient knowledge. Fracastoro built on existing notions by adding a "compatible truth." The environment and living conditions became potential players in disease spread and perpetuation in a way that was still unclear but more palpable. Movement became relevant too, as did proximity between people and sources of infection, and poverty and hygiene. Fracastoro broke down disease into new components, with each one of his original "proposed additional truths" complementing pre-existing theories.

Although he proposed this paradigm shift, Fracastoro was unable to completely eradicate the ancient Galenic model of how disease spread. This would only happen much later. The final push came from the efforts of two other Italian doctors, Francesco Redi (1626–1698) and Lazzaro Spallanzani (1729–1799), and later the endeavors of Louis Pasteur (1822–1895).

But why did it take so long?

Fracastoro's theory lacked many elements and clashed with existing knowledge. Plus, one major piece of the puzzle was still missing: microorganisms. This seems difficult to imagine nowadays as we can look through electron microscopes or use other similar technologies to visualize invisible nature. But consider this: we're talking about creatures that are living and reproducing inside us. Unimaginable at the time. Back then, there was always the fear of attracting unwanted attention from religious authorities or worse still, the Inquisition. This certainly hindered creative thought.

And how did we get to actually see this microcosm within us?

By pure chance. As disruptive as a basketball smashing through a glass window. The revolution was caused by an unwitting scientist who actually had little or nothing to do with medicine or science. Antonie van Leeuwenhoek (1632–1723) was a Dutch optician and naturalist who made history by being the first to observe microorganisms through a microscope. Thanks to his studies he exposed us to a universe which until then had been invisible. As if by magic, we had proof of a plethora of living organisms that were imperceptible to the naked eye, but which could finally be seen thanks to the power of magnifying lenses.

How did Antonie van Leeuwenhoek become the first "microscopist"?

Incredibly, the world of microbes was discovered thanks to a push in the right direction from a totally different scientific field. For his research, van Leeuwenhoek relied on the great advances of the seventeenth century in the construction of optical lenses, the work of Galileo Galilei and his contemporaries. But the game changer was that van Leeuwenhoek focused on a different scale. While Galileo used lenses to observe celestial bodies, large and distant, the Dutch entrepreneur-scientist used them to explore the minuscule.

That's really surprising, if you think that he didn't start out as a scientist.

Actually, van Leeuwenhoek became a scientist thanks to learning-by-doing: he never really studied and didn't come from the scientific and cultural establishment of the time. But it just goes to show, creativity will flourish anywhere and will always find its way. He was a true NL.

He came from the Netherlands, but what was his job?

He started out as an accountant in a draper's shop. Being very good at his job, he eventually set up his own business selling luxury textiles and trimmings. But beyond his nose for business, he also had the curiosity that inspires a true genius. Our NL was intrigued by the details of the materials, enchanted by the softness of velvets and silks. He wanted to go beyond what his fingertips could feel and understand the differences in fabrics beyond touch. He wanted to see the details with his own eyes and it may even have become a sort of obsession for him. This is how his career as a scientist began: he wanted to see more, so he turned to lenses and tapped their extraordinary potential. He taught himself how to build microscopes, and was finally able to observe more clearly the innate characteristics of his wares. During his lifetime he went on to craft around 500 lenses and build dozens of microscopes (which he guarded jealously, never showing them to anyone), using candles and mirrors to increase their functionality.

Those lenses and microscopes would unveil a new universe (for us too).

Van Leeuwenhoek, initially just a very curious businessman, discovered what is truly another dimension. We could compare it to the future discovery of a mechanism for activating telepathy, for example. The miracle of magnification revealed a previously unknown, and otherwise invisible – but totally real – world, one that coexisted with us and within us. This new "micro-world" was extremely diverse. It contained everything from tadpoles to red-blood cells to capillaries and muscle fibers. (Yes – incredibly – an accountant was the first person to discover the detail of capillaries and muscle fibers!) For a moment, imagine the wonder! Van Leeuwenhoek started off wanting to examine velvets and silk, and ended up discovering a universe. One can imagine how his curiosity grew into an expanding spiral of self-perceived omnipotence: he couldn't stop magnifying everything he came across. A true serial magnifier.

How did the scientific community come to hear of his discoveries?

Van Leeuwenhoek had an intelligent, generous friend, a physician named Reinier de Graaf (1641–1673). He was the one who brought van Leeuwenhoek's work to the attention of the Royal Society in London, which in 1673 published a letter from the Dutch optician in which he described what he had seen through his microscopes: molds, bees and lice. He had also used his powerful lenses on virtually everything within his reach: gunpowder, sperm, blood cells, coffee beans, minerals, even going so far as to identify a parasite, Giardia, in his own feces. He knew that with his invention (which he was extremely proud and protective of) he had made it possible to reveal an almost infinite number of parallel worlds populated by every form of life and matter. He wrote numerous letters to the Royal Society in which he described his wondrous findings: an insect's compound eye and its stinger, the intricate lamellate structure of wood. All with illustrations drawn by hand and detailed notes of his observations. These reports came as a single copy (with no backup), sent by a horseback courier from Delft in the Netherlands all the way across the sea to London.

His voyages through the micro-universe led him to yet another incredible discovery. Van Leeuwenhoek, observing a droplet of water from a lake, saw moving particles. That was the moment when the invisible world he'd discovered became alive. Alive and kicking!

A double discovery.

Minuscule creatures shaped a bit like tiny slippers were moving on their own, so they looked like animals, even if they were incredibly small. Which is why he named them *diertgens*, "small animals," later translated to the Latin *animalcula* and in English *animalcule*. That universe which he'd just unveiled was full of living, moving organisms which turned out to be essential for life and death on Earth.

How did the scientific establishment react at the time?

Initially, the Royal Society was skeptical of the discoveries made by the now de facto Dutch naturalist. Van Leeuwenhoek had to travel to London, and after the visit of three delegates representing the English institution witnessed one of his demonstrations, the conceptual roadmap to the idea that microorganisms could in fact exist was drawn. Antonie van Leeuwenhoek was elected to the Royal Society in February 1680. Although he never attended a Royal Society meeting (he was too busy enjoying his newly-won fame throughout Europe), he considered it a great honor.

We will never know if he lost his mind in the immensity of the new world he had revealed. A sane person who made such a dramatic breakthrough would want to tell the world, and share the thrill of the revolutionary discovery. Regrettably van Leeuwenhoek took most of his secrets to the grave (lenses and microscopes included)... and that really is a dissonant behavior that never helps society to move forward for the greater good.

Knowledge is built on the work of others. If everyone behaved with this in mind, we wouldn't have to start from scratch each and every time someone wanted to explore a new idea. We'd still be painting in caves. This also reminds me of an aphorism attributed to Bernard of Chartres, later reformulated by Newton: "We are like dwarfs sitting on the shoulders of giants. We see more, and see things that are more distant, not because our sight is superior or because we are taller than they were, but because they offer us a higher perspective as their great stature adds to ours." This is an important lesson which we should reflect on more often if we want to benefit from all the scientific progress of the past.

You often mention transversality and cross-fertilization of knowledge. How are these concepts relevant in this case?

Well, it's obvious! Here we have a scientific discovery of revolutionary scope brought about by a businessman. Someone who had to account for and verify everything with his own eyes rather than dedicate his life to abstract concepts. Van Leeuwenhoek initially used his microscope not for medical or scientific purposes but for his own economic interests: he wanted to understand textiles in more detail so that he could improve his business. But the extraordinary part of this unique and bizarre story was that he had such an open mind that he discovered a universe which had little to do with fabrics, ribbons, and lace. And despite uncertainties and reluctance, the scientific world of that time was ready to explore new horizons that would lead to unimaginable innovations. It was a question of someone being in the right place at the right time.

Notes

[1] The word "miasma" derives from the ancient Greek μίασμα, "contamination," a term which shares the same root as the verb μιαίνειν, "besmirch," "contaminate." In ancient Greek medicine, beginning with Hippocrates, miasma came to denote a noxious exhalation, specifically those emanating from corpses and stagnant waters. These vapors were believed to be the cause of diseases such as malaria, infections and contagions.

[2] The word "virus" derives from the Latin noun *virus*, meaning "slimy liquid," "poison." It was only from the sixteenth century onwards that this term entered permanently into medical jargon, to describe an infectious pus. At the end of the nineteenth century the word began to be used to denote a newly discovered infectious agent, smaller than bacteria.

−2 Discovering the Unthinkable

So let's recap what you've been saying. At this point we've landed on a new truth – they probably even thought it was fake news back then. We now have visible proof that diseases aren't caused by odors but by poisons that contain deadly miniscule particles. What a leap forward!

And not only that. We also realized that these poisons were contagious, because they could spread to other susceptible organisms. They were made up of tiny micro-organisms that by a lucky coincidence appeared before the eyes of a textile merchant – not a scientist! – as he peered through his microscope. Van Leeuwenhoek had discovered a Universe that was so big that nobody would believe him at first. For this and many other reasons it took nearly 200 years to reach any kind of consensus around certain pathogens. And this was just the beginning.

Identifying the agents of disease was one thing – defending ourselves against viruses and bacteria was a completely different story. The very notion of "active defense" was not an easy one to imagine. The idea of protecting yourself from something invisible is nearly impossible to conceive, much less comprehend. How can you fight something that you can't see? Well, to continue on with our story, it was almost one hundred years after van Leeuwenhoek's discoveries that a British physician and naturalist, Edward Jenner (1749–1823), introduced the practice of vaccination.

The first vaccine was developed to combat smallpox: one of the deadliest diseases.

Smallpox is another so-called "plague" which disfigures faces, maims bodies and souls, and disrupts social systems by decimating entire populations. Notwithstanding its deadly potential, it has one positive characteristic: it is a fairly simple enemy. Science has come to know smallpox well because it acts like a conventional virus and obeys fundamental rules which are easy to recognize and understand. In a sense, smallpox behaves itself.

At the time of its discovery, it was really a question of figuring out certain mechanisms which today seem pretty simple. Smallpox is a killer, a disease which brings you face to face with death. But we could call it a gentleman killer – if you survive it once, it will never be able to hurt you again. And this was already clear in Jenner's time. In fact, some practitioners in the East had already invented a procedure to provoke small controlled infections which could act as a protection against natural exposure. This process was known as *variolation*.

Wasn't Jenner the father of immunization?

Yes and no. There are reports of a preventative therapy against smallpox practiced by the Circassians, who lived in the North Caucasus (now a part of the Russian Federation). They noticed that smallpox occurred only once in a lifetime, so they deliberately exposed their children to the virus to establish a very mild, localized infection which could protect them for the rest of their lives. The Turks adopted a similar practice, which became a standard in the city of Constantinople. In England, the voluntary grafting of smallpox was introduced thanks to the work of Emmanuel Timoni (1670–1718), a physician, and the foresight of Lady Mary Wortley Montagu (1689–1762). Together with her husband, the ambassador to Constantinople, she had observed the benefits of variolation directly. She was so convinced of its effectiveness that she decided to apply it to her own children. Similar techniques had also been used for centuries in the Ionian Islands, in Istria and in the regions bordering Greece, harking all the way back to possible origins in Venice and even as far away as China.

You mentioned Lady Mary Wortley Montagu. Do we finally have a female character in our story?

Yes! Lady Mary is the first woman mentioned in this story and deserves special attention. By introducing smallpox variolation in England, she played a very prominent role in the history of Western health, although, sadly, she has rarely been recognized for her achievements. She was a brave woman who travelled widely, as we can see from the many letters she wrote over the years. These letters brought her visibility, but with it, harsh criticism with regard to her freedom of thought and personal life.

In her correspondence she describes a life that sounds like a classic romance: she was passionate about writing from an early age; she married against her father's will; ascended into English political and intellectual society; lived in Constantinople as the wife of the British Ambassador. There she learned about variolation against smallpox and exported it back to England. Some of her letters revealed quite a few details about her private life (including her affairs). Amongst the personal and professional challenges Lady Mary faced were the cultural restrictions of her time. But despite these, she was able to bring a very innovative protective practice to people in need and that's what we remember her for. It's true, as was often case during those times, that the roles women played in history were overlooked. But today we fully acknowledge Lady Mary Montagu as a pioneer in the advancement of immunization.

I wonder if a form of the anti-vaccination lobby existed back then.

It certainly did. There are actually some very interesting attempts to reject vaccination including documented forms of propaganda. An example advertisement from the 1860's suggests rather strongly to the reader that some sectors of society felt that vaccination was exactly a good idea.

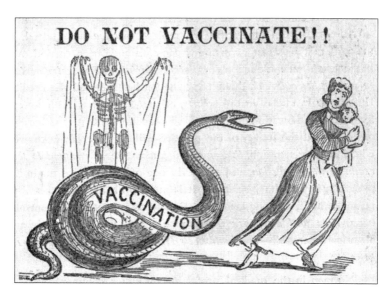

Anti-vaccination cartoon from the *Scrapbook of Anti-Vaccinations Clippings*, 1890s. Courtesy of the Historical Medical Library of The College of Physicians of Philadelphia.

How did variolation – a rather rudimental approach at the time – come to be accepted?

What's interesting about this story is that the practice of controlled inoculation using infectious material was established via personal reports from people with little in the way of a formal education. It was through witnessing the effectiveness directly and sharing the news by word-of-mouth that it became widespread throughout Europe as a practice, overcoming linguistic, religious, and cultural barriers. It gained traction for one simple reason: it worked. The "wondrous graft," as described in an Italian poem from the eighteenth century tells us that inoculation was indeed seen as something close to a miracle, encircled in a halo of magic. Such a reputation gives any public health procedure a huge advantage, as it is accepted and welcomed by all classes of society. Effectively it "goes viral." Variolation was instrumental in engaging the poorest, the farthest-flung (those living in villages and remote rural areas), the illiterate as well as the educated – all fearful of a disease that until then had always left a deep and visible scar on society.

If variolation worked, why didn't they just stick with that? Why was there a need for another procedure and why was vaccination different?

These "controlled infections" provoked by variolation were dangerous and far from standardized. They did provide some protection, but they could also do great damage or even cause death if there was an adverse reaction. So variolation was a solution, but certainly not an adequate one in terms of temporary and effective procedural safety. Something better had to be found.

And this is where Jenner comes in.

Exactly. Jenner was an observer and a "connector of dots." He noticed that in addition to the survivors of natural infection and those treated with variolation, there was another group of people who also appeared to be immune to smallpox: milkmaids. But not all milkmaids, only those who had been previously contaminated by an ugly hand infection which came from contact with similar-looking lesions on the cows' udders. What distinguished these two groups of workers? There was still another piece missing from the puzzle.

Here is where his game-changing idea comes in. He understood that a "related" virus, even if it came from another species (it had to be an animal), could provide clinical protection against smallpox. A breakthrough intuition which opened a previously invisible door, the port of entry into a new world: immunology.

In point of fact, Jenner didn't get there first though. In 1774 another British physician, Benjamin Jesty (1736–1816), had "vaccinated" his entire family with cowpox virus and prevented the disease. But he never wrote up his findings or made them public, which is likely the reason why he missed out on the lion's share of the scientific recognition and glory. In a similar vein to van

Leeuwenhoek with his microscopes, he failed to properly inform the scientific community of what he had discovered.

And Jenner did.

In 1798 in the form of a letter to his friend Caleb Hillier Parry (1755–1822), and at his own expense, Jenner published *An Inquiry into Causes and Effects of the Variolae Vaccinae*. To him, this seemed to be the only way to get his findings into the public domain since the Royal Society had shown no interest in his work. His revolutionary discoveries and intuition clashed violently with the existing dogmas of the time. The far-fetched idea that a human disease could be avoided with a pre-emptive dose of infected matter obtained from an animal was just too extreme, not to mention disgusting. It clearly went beyond existing boundaries.

This is an incredible story which offers several clear examples of how the best science works. Jenner's discovery shattered taboos, questioned dogmas, broke down barriers, and was powerfully disruptive and uncompromising. His number one conclusion was that a disease lethal to humans, smallpox, could be prevented. This prevention could be achieved by exposing susceptible individuals to infected material collected from lesions found on the udders of dairy cows affected by a disease called Cowpox. Conclusion number two had a very pragmatic consequence. It solved the problem of product availability since it could also be obtained from cows that had been deliberately infected. These points combined to produce a key discovery: heterologous vaccines – i.e. those made from an agent that is different from the agent you are trying to protect against. He was generating protection from smallpox through cowpox, a disease which can be transmitted from animals to humans. All this had an enormous clinical impact in the efforts to save humanity from one of its worst afflictions. Jenner effectively scored three times with a single shot. And he did so by envisioning a connection between animal and human health.

And almost as if to ensure that future generations – including our own – wouldn't forget the fundamental link between human and animal health, Dr. Jenner adopted the term vaccine (from the Latin *vacca*, cow). A term that over time has extended beyond its original meaning to indicate a preparation which can be administered to an organism to stimulate the production of specific defenses. In other words, a generator of active immunity.

Jenner would explore this idea further over the next three years. His publications (*Further Observations on the Variolae Vaccinae*, *A Continuation of Facts and Observations relative to the Variolae Vaccinae* and *The Origin of the Vaccine Inoculation*), would leave an indelible mark on the history of medicine and the overall approach to public health management.

Jenner's revolution challenged and overturned the theories of the time, and was quickly recognized internationally: his works were translated as early as 1799. But his discoveries left his colleagues of the Royal Society in total dismay especially as his ideas clashed violently with the distinction and separation between species, particularly between animals and human beings.

Admittedly, it seems almost absurd.

That's right. Initially, Jenner's ideas were so innovative that they were rejected for being "too revolutionary." And Jenner's contemporaries had a point. Just try to put yourself in their shoes: somebody suggests infected material obtained from a sick animal can be used to protect humans from getting sick? Cross-protection? It sounds less like science and more like science fiction, but that's exactly how it worked. The solution that introduced vaccination to the world had been hidden on cows' udders for centuries. It's a classic case of hiding in plain sight.

Yet another example of a revolution due to an unexpected crossover.

Yes, yes, yes. The universe of microbiology was discovered by a textile merchant; the concept of disease spread was developed by a doctor-philosopher-astronomer who had many intuitions, but remained entangled between the old and the new (still partially convinced that celestial bodies could have some impact on health). And then a heretical revolution, especially as far as the relationship between humans and animals, was introduced by Jenner. The pillars of microbiology were progressively defined and deciphered thanks to incursions and observations that originated for the most part in other fields. The subject was embraced by revolutionary thinkers with visions unbiased by prejudice. They were ready to stand behind their own ideas even if they contradicted mainstream opinion and institutions of the period. Who knows, maybe most of them were NL, at least in their mindset.

Here we go again with NL. But what does it mean?

We'll get to that eventually, don't worry.

So, after Jenner's discoveries with the expansion of vaccination, can we finally start fighting viruses and bacteria?

Once again, yes and no. The first attempts at vaccination were successful, but there was still an awfully long way to go. The next building block towards constructing a more complete theory explaining the nature of infectious diseases could have come from the animal world or from the environment. For the time being, the idea that disease transmission occurred by virtue of an almost "magical" malignant force was still widespread.

Rather than some sort of "micro-world," it seems they were looking at a sea of unknowns.

Nailed it! Of course, a new world is full of unknowns. Scientists were hunting for invisible creatures. A new world that had to be conceived and imagined. And were these creatures harmful or beneficial? Were they mobile or stationary? Were they rod-shaped or round? Bacteria and viruses are everywhere, in people who are healthy as well as those who are sick: it became necessary to understand how to classify this new jungle that was gradually emerging.

As a virologist who benefitted from this historical work, I feel I should acknowledge the thousands of microbiologists who over the centuries spent countless hours bent over microscopes trying to figure out patterns, in an attempt to classify what they were seeing. Their work provided the bedrock of understanding upon which we have based the study of infectious disease. They often took some considerable risks: imagine working at a time when you had no idea if the agent you were growing was harmful. What if you decided that to understand what a certain pathogen did? You had to expose an animal to it and see what happened. This is how the first animal experiments began.

Quick digression: there's a lot of debate today about this last issue… animal testing.

As far as the ethical debate is concerned, as a trained veterinarian, I am clearly concerned with animal health and welfare. In this context, all I can say is that animal experimentation has served a fundamental role in advancing the understanding of human and animal health. The scientific community has dramatically reduced the number of animals used in testing in recent years. And rightly so. Handling procedures and experimental protocols are also strictly regulated. Unfortunately, there are still some studies that we can perform only on animals. In the future, big data-based observations will support further improvements in animal welfare and a lower dependence upon animal use in critical experiments.

And so, another leap to the nineteenth century, the era of science and technology.

During the course of the nineteenth century our knowledge of health, began to organize in a more structured way. Almost like the colored Lego bricks of our childhood. A process of reorganization triggered convergence and consolidation, merging the discoveries made in multiple fields. And we know today that the fundamental pillars of medicine were erected from the assembly of centuries of scattered rocks of knowledge. But the critical mass of information that was discovered needed to be re-structured completely, as simple add-ons to the old framework were no longer feasible. At this stage, biomedical disciplines could finally begin to take a different, more appropriate shape. Like a three-dimensional puzzle made of irregular pieces, the knowledge was assembled at first in a somewhat haphazard fashion: a plethora of inventions, intuitions, experiments, tests and checks, scribbles and sketches which little by little found reciprocal support and corroboration. Science had become a new language which could promote progress and improve health more than ever before. A collective work of herculean proportions which required Vesalius' anatomic tables, to discover an entire parallel universe inhabited by series of microscopic creatures of efficient shapes progressively identified as cocci, bacilli, vibrios… And we haven't even mentioned the role parasites have in the interchange yet.

In other words, knowledge pertaining to health was driven to become increasingly vertical, more focused, as scholars delved deeper into each topic to gain a more complete understanding. The nineteenth century became the time of a truly colossal transformation: "the cell theory" developed by Rudolf Virchow (1821–1902) definitively buried the humoral theory which had dominated medical science debate for more than two thousand years. This was followed by an endless series of successive breakthroughs. Louis Pasteur (1822–1895) and Robert Koch (1843–1910) identified the mysterious and invisible causes of numerous and deadly infectious diseases. The use of ether for anesthesia opened the door to the miracles of surgery, while x-rays allowed us to see the insides of our bodies from the outside, in a ghost-like clarity.

Does this new verticalized framework also include microbiology?

Microbiology was one of the major drivers that pushed the ancient doctrine governing health and illness over the cliff's edge.

From a virologist's perspective the humoral theory was shaken by observing the dynamics of disease transmission, which required mechanisms that it could never foresee or accommodate. Disease transmission required the development of the concept of *seminaria*, a possible mechanism for pathogen propagation, and finally the identification of the characteristics of the suspected agents. The casual intrusion of a cloth merchant playing with lenses shattered a conceptual framework which had dominated the field of medicine for over twenty centuries. The works of Galen and Pasteur not only occurred in different eras but were also based on completely different sources of information; they could not be reconciled.

Years of dramatic clashes between old and new factions resulted in persecution and violence that were, to differing extents, directed against the innovators. Nevertheless, there was a move towards a new paradigm that still preserved the original vision: circularity. Indeed, with the advent of microbiology, circularity was enhanced and expanded.

What do you mean by circularity in the context of microbiology?

Microbes became the new link between separate worlds. They are perfectly fitted to take on the role of connectors between the health of humans, animals, and plants. Today this circularity is made even more obvious by contemporary challenges, such as the issue of antibiotic resistance. Super-killer microbes, evolving throughout decades of antibiotic treatment, are the result of bacterial circulation and re-circulation between humans and their surroundings. Domestic animals can act as a source of infection, as can the environment. Just think of the infections you can pick up in a hospital: you're admitted for a standard surgical procedure and risk contracting a lethal infection from your new surroundings, where instead you were actually hoping to be cured.

How does this microbiological revolution begin?

The consensus of scientists is that this begins with Pasteur, a restless, passionate man. During his life he was fully dedicated to the impossible mission of exploring the world "beyond the lens," with a distinctly NL approach: open, candid, and receptive.

NL again, does it have something to do with the Netherlands? Are you referring to the Dutchman again?

Just bear with me a bit longer. What's essential now is that with Pasteur we gain a more detailed and in-depth view of what was previously invisible. The parallel universe that van Leeuwenhoek (yes, the Dutchman) had only peered into briefly. This micro-universe has coexisted with us since the beginning in silence, except when conditions made it either dangerous or extremely beneficial for health.

Pasteur was a chemist, and he was a particularly good one too: always questioning, always investigating. His acumen drew him to the most urgent and significant problems of that time for agriculture and animal husbandry. He was a pragmatic scientist who wasn't afraid of engaging with concrete (and very thorny) problems which had substantial repercussions for both the economy and society in general.

What was the practical impact of his research?

Huge. He was a true pioneer in many fields. Just think of pasteurization, the procedure which bears his name. Today it brings to mind the milk we buy at the supermarket, but actually, Pasteur originally developed a thermal treatment to "cure wine diseases": a way to avoid excessive fermentation. Only later would it become clear that this process could also be used with other perishable products such as milk and beer. By applying heat to food, Pasteur obtained two results: he was able to slow down deterioration, and he eliminated several bacteria that were harmful to human health. If you think that's not a big accomplishment, just consider that three of Pasteur's children died of typhoid. He had experienced the effects of unwanted contaminants at a very personal level.

Pasteur also invented vaccines against two dreaded diseases of the time which were dangerous to both livestock and humans. He experimented with the *anthrax bacillus* (*B. anthracis*), producing a thermally-treated vaccine which proved effective. Ambitious ingenuity led him to develop vaccines against rabies, an incurable disease which always led to death after excruciating suffering. Rabies could be contracted after a bite or contact with the saliva of an infected animal, be it a bat, a dog, or a Bengal tiger. It was a tremendous health issue at the time. And he worked it out.

Were other scientists active in the same area at that time?

He wasn't alone. In this phase Pasteur collaborated with colleagues Émile Roux (1853–1933), Joseph-Henri Toussaint (1847–1890) and Robert Koch to break down the barriers separating human and animal health. It was clear that animals and humans could contract the same disease, and this observation led to novel areas of research. Pasteur understood that chemical substances or physical forces (such as heat) could interact with the "invisible world" neutralizing some of its more harmful effects. All of a sudden, thanks to the creativity of a chemist, the study of microbes in animal models became a resource for the study of human health: two universes that had appeared separate for many centuries were joined again, and more closely than ever before.

A super-achiever as a chemist.

That's why you should never draw boundaries around professions. Pasteur was trained as a chemist but he was undoubtedly much more. He was a scientist with a flexible and challenging mind. As a result of his work and of that of his peers, by the end of the nineteenth century a new scientific era dawned. Bacteriology became the key to unlocking essential concepts and merging the boundaries between human, animal, plant and environmental health.

A new road which leads us to modern times.

One step at a time these innovators paved the way to our current level of knowledge. But a major breakthrough was still required. A breakthrough which in some respects was even more astonishing. Not only were certain microscopic and macroscopic parasites transmissible from animals to humans and vice versa, some of them could also use a third organism as a "shuttle" to move from one host to another. A new frontier of knowledge opened up: diseases transmitted by vectors,[1] so-called "hitchhiking" pathogens.

Can you give us an example?

Malaria is still the most important one. Since ancient times, it had been a veritable scourge of populations living in tropical and sub-tropical marshlands the world over. The Italian word malaria (from *mal'aria* "noxious or harmful air") gives a better idea of its essential characteristics than the French word *paludisme*. It suggests that infection was evaporating from stagnant marsh waters, and was indeed considered by the ancients to be the cause of the disease. Malaria is to some extent connected to bad air, but clearly this is not the cause. Instead, the cause of malaria is linked to mosquitoes that live in swampy, still-air environments.

But at that time two fundamental links were missing: the identification of the *seminaria* or the *animalcula* responsible for the disease (in the case of malaria, a comma-shaped protozoa); and the knowledge that the disease could be transmitted by a vector (another organism that carried the malarial protozoa from host to host). This is critical because it means that our little comma-shaped protozoal "creature" is incapable of moving from an infected person to a healthy one without help. When it needs a ride from a helper, this helper has to transform it and carry it on to its next host. Think of it like this: our comma needs to change into a full stop before it can generate new sentences (infections). And where does this transformation take place? In a mosquito's gut. Only when it has matured from comma to full stop, inside the stomach of an annoying insect, is it ready to attack another host. No mosquitoes means no infection and therefore no disease. Not exactly easy to understand.

How did the systematic study of malaria begin?

It didn't really originate from a strong scientific interest, but for economic reasons. Both the English and the French felt the impact of malaria in their colonies, and the disease was also endemic in Italy at that time. An Italian doctor named Giovanni Battista Grassi (1854–1925) made a significant impact on the understanding of malaria.

Why is that? What was Grassi's background before he started to research malaria?

He graduated with a degree in medicine from the University of Pavia, and was a highly active researcher. After university, he devoted himself to research in the fields of biology and zoology, and became a visiting scholar in various European institutes: he studied the eel's reproductive cycle, discovered a new species of Arachnid and named it after his wife (*Koenenia mirabilis*). He also described termite societies in a series of seminal works.

What led him to study malaria and mosquitoes?

A rather unrelated perspective, as usual. In 1888 Grassi began studying malaria in birds, together with the medical clinician Riccardo Feletti. In 1890 they published a monograph in which they described their observations, focusing on malaria in the owl, the pigeon, and the sparrow. Grassi was a curious man, and beyond studying birds he was totally fascinated by insects and taxonomy.[2] He had a penchant for collecting and cataloging. And he was really good at it. So much so that in 1896 he won one of the most important acknowledgments in the field of biology (the Royal Society's Darwin Medal) for his contributions to entomology and marine biology.

So, what was his contribution to combatting malaria?

Although an Englishman and Nobel laureate, Ronald Ross, is credited with discovering that malaria is transmitted by mosquitoes, Grassi played a major role in our understanding of the disease. He realized that mosquitoes were involved, but he also knew very well that not all mosquitoes are the same. His taxonomy background taught him that there were major differences between species, and that is was highly likely that not all species of mosquito could transmit malaria. To demonstrate that the "shuttle" for infection was the *Anopheles* mosquito, he conducted a clinical experiment with a single volunteer, a brave man named Mr. Sola, who agreed to sleep for 30 nights in a room infested with mosquitoes taken from an endemic area and therefore presumably carrying malaria. None of that first set of mosquitoes were *Anopheles* species, and sure enough, Mr. Sola didn't contract the disease. Mr. Sola then agreed to be involved in a second experiment. Grassi released some recently-collected *Anopheles* mosquitoes into the same room and within a few days poor Mr. Sola began to shake and shiver, developing a high fever. It was malaria. Grassi had just closed a circle within a circle.

Notes

[1] "Vector" comes from the Latin vector "conductor, carrier," deriving from the verb *vehĕre*, "conduct, carry." In epidemiology, this term refers to hematophagous animals (i.e. blood feeders) such as fleas, ticks, mosquitoes, bats etc. These creatures can transmit, via a sting or a bite, infectious diseases.

[2] Taxonomy (from the Greek τάξις, *taxis*, "order," and νόμος, *nomos*, "rule" or "law") is the quintessential "discipline of classification." Generally, the word indicates biological taxonomy, which is a system of criteria by which organisms are classified in a hierarchy of grouped taxa.

−1   Finding Hidden Truths

With the discovery of microbes and protozoa, we can fast-forward to modern times. Right?

With the discovery and study of microbes on one hand, and clinical cases on the other, great progress was made in our knowledge and understanding of certain disease-related mechanisms. Clearly, with each step forward the scenario and possible interactions became more complicated. Malaria and its bizarre cycle was just one such example. Between the nineteenth and twentieth centuries there was an acceleration, with many of the discoveries and findings being gathered together and assembled into a more complete story. The reconstruction gained speed. But we needed a bird's eye view to get a broader perspective in order to finally bring the ever-expanding picture truly into focus.

Where do we start?

Do you like Game of Thrones?

The books or the series? And wait, what does GoT have to do with it?

Well, the story we're telling is also a saga, much more consequential and in some respects more engaging than the award-winning TV series. Of course, our heroes in this case aren't young warriors with long, disheveled hair but mature, balding scientists. The name of John Snow (1813--1858), an English physician and scientist, for instance, sounds just like Jon Snow, Lord Commander of the Night's Watch. We really don't know if George R. R. Martin, author of the bestselling books, had any intention of drawing a parallel. In any event, behind his ordinary and perhaps slightly sad appearance, even John (with an 'h', the doctor) is a revolutionary, and in his own way a hero. The first of nine children (a very challenging way to grow up in any era), and fortunately from a family that was comfortably well-off, John studied medicine and became an anesthesiologist and obstetrician, presiding over the birth of two of Queen Victoria's children. He could have gone on to a successful career as a clinician but instead his life took a different turn.

In what way was he revolutionary?

In 1854, London was hit by a tragic and relentless cholera epidemic: within a few days hundreds of people fell ill and died. Nobody knew what to do. Indeed, no one at the time understood the causes of the disease: the miasma theory was still very popular and, among the *animalcula* frenetically being classified, there was no microbe (yet) which could be related causally to cholera. With perfect timing and remarkable intuition, Snow realized that all the cholera cases had something in common. From his shelves he pulled out an instrument which until then had been almost entirely overlooked in health-related disciplines, introducing a new dimension to the study of disease.

What instrument was that?

A map. The revolutionary idea was to mark the progress of the disease on a map of London.

Is that it?

Many things appear obvious... once someone else has pointed them out. Today mapping a disease is one of the first things we do: it may seem trivial, but it's actually ingenious. Snow knew that to understand the epidemic, and in doing so stop it, he needed a new "filter," which would sift through the information coming from the outbreaks. To use the modern term, he began to geo-localize cases of cholera on a map of Soho, in London. And so, Epidemiology was born: a discipline which focuses on neither the patient nor the source of disease, but on the dynamics of how it spreads.

And along with the insight of "moving diseases" comes the notion of prevention. If it moves, it can be stopped – even if we ignore the cause. It doesn't much matter whether it's cholera or salmonella: what's important is understanding how to break the chain of transmission. This idea brings together a whole set of different skills (not purely medical), for example organizational skills in terms of procedures and communication, as well as cartography.

And to what conclusion did John Snow come?

That the water supply for all the homes of almost all the people who had gotten sick or died from cholera came from one specific pump, in Broad Street. With the help of the Reverend Henry Whitehead, who was quite doubtful of the theory, Snow convinced the local authorities to close the pump. The story goes that on that same night all the cholera deaths stopped.

A success story!

Well, not really. Even though he was a physician of a certain stature, it wasn't easy for him to influence public opinion as to the origin of the illness. Snow must have been rather confused. He was particularly skeptical about the "miasma theory," which prevailed at the time and which still held that epidemics such as cholera were caused by a dangerous form of "bad air."

On the other hand, in those years the germ theory hadn't been widely accepted, so Snow ignored the specific mechanism that could actually transmit the disease. The facts led him to believe that the spread of cholera was not caused by fetid air, but instead the contamination of the water supply due to sewage leaks. He had initially proposed his theory in 1849 in a treatise called *On the Mode of Communication of Cholera*, which was published for a second time in 1855, with far more in-depth research on the role of the water supply during the London epidemic of 1854.

So, disease spreads not only through air and insects, but also through water.

Yes. This was quite a substantial breakthrough, because water is tangible. You can feel it, you can touch it. Water is much more visible and traceable than air. In Snow's hypothesis, water replaces vanishing miasma. Water also has a symbolic meaning. It's not just the element which covers over 70% of the Earth's surface. The environment is water, and water is the environment – soaking it, penetrating it, hydrating it and giving it life. Water surrounds us in oceans, lakes, and ponds. We are made of water; it runs through our body, we drink it and we eliminate it. Snow's great discovery was a revolutionary development in the medical wisdom of the time, taking that wisdom to a whole new level. And this leads us to reflect back centuries to Hippocrates' intuition that human health was also dependent on the health of water. (If you look closely, you'll see the word *aqua* in the lower part of the diagram on this book's front cover.)

So, we're back to circles, the idea of environment as an "influencer" on health and disease.

The role of the environment, which was one of the founding principles of the humoral theory, finally began to expand conceptually and acquire a solid scientific basis.

Water isn't just a vehicle for infections and parasites: the temperature of water can have profound consequences (think of coral bleaching, the ice melting, the rising sea levels). Water contains chemical substances; creatures inhabit it, from the microscopic to the gigantic. John Snow found that the source of the deadly London cholera epidemic was linked to water, solving the problem in an exemplary and functional way. And surprisingly the mystery was solved without ever identifying the culprit. In reality, it would take another thirty years for *Vibrio cholerae* to be formally identified, with the meticulous and analytical work of the German scientist Robert Koch.

It looks like the early microbiologists kept themselves very busy.

That's right, and there was a lot to do. For thousands of years humans had been at the mercy of microbes: already in the thirteenth century B.C.E. Chinese texts documented the fear that the outbreak of an infectious disease could induce. According to estimates, the Black Death of 1347–1352 was responsible for the annihilation of at least a third of the European population. Its consequences were far-reaching: the plague triggered an upheaval of the habits and customs of the period, even calling into question religion in the process. The dreaded disease brought with it so much pain and desperation that people lost all sense of direction and purpose. Nothing made sense in the face of death spread by the plague's relentless march.

Who would have thought back then that the plague is generally transmitted by a flea? And where did the flea pick up this nasty infection? From a rat. So, the plague jumps from animals to humans thanks to a flea (one of nature's best jumpers: if they were the size of a human, they could jump just about as high as the Empire State Building). This is how plague spreads. Infection circulates in rats, so all you need is one infected rat. A flea bites the rat and becomes infected, then jumps and lands on a human, bites him, and the human gets sick. So once again, we have a human disease which originates from an animal infection and which depends on the state of the environment (filthy or clean). The lesson here is clear: it's better not to live within jumping range of a flea, and generally speaking, rats are to be avoided altogether.

By the way, when do hygiene and cleanliness enter the story?

What was truly revolutionary was the antiseptic method developed by Joseph Lister (1827–1912), who was called "one of mankind's greatest benefactors" by the German pathologist Virchow. And he wasn't exaggerating, if you consider that the introduction of Lister's hygienic practices literally saved millions of lives.

In what way?

Lister, a Scotsman, was a professor of surgery at the University of Glasgow. He read Pasteur's studies on fermentation, and became convinced that something similar to the fermentation process in yeast occurred in wounds too.

Where does his insight lie?

He realized that infections in wounds could be caused or transmitted from patient to patient through microbes. Further, he suspected that these microbes were living on the hands of the doctors handling the patients. At this point, Lister began to think of ways to break the infectious cycle inside hospital wards. As a side note, in those days standards of personal hygiene were generally poor, and the importance of hygiene was not fully understood.

This lack of awareness led to dramatic consequences, especially for patients undergoing surgery; often the damage done by infection was worse than the benefit gained from the operation. Any operation was itself already hard enough. Imagine invasive surgery after being given only basic anesthesia, essentially with no diagnostic points of reference (there was no diagnostic imaging), no sterile surgical tools and no antibiotics. If you didn't die from the operation, you often died in the aftermath.

This was the reality of the day. But Lister was convinced that post-operatory infections could be prevented or at least inhibited by acting on the medical and paramedical personnel, on the surgical instruments and on patients themselves. A multi-level strategy converging around the goal of destroying the microbes that cause post-operatory infections, septicemia and gangrene. And guess how he got the idea?

I can see a potential transversal insight coming here.

It came to him, in perfect NL style, from observing a practice which occurs to this day in livestock farming all over the world. To recirculate nutrients into the soil, fields are irrigated with sewage, creating another form of the human-animal-environment connection.

Human health is the result of multiple drivers; you can't think of it in terms of boxed off compartments: within the biosphere, everything is connected. We have to accept it: as humans, we are not programmed to live separately from other living beings. And more importantly, we can't, even if we try.

But what did Lister actually observe?

He noticed that in the city of Carlisle, the sewage was treated with phenol (an antiseptic) before being spread over the fields. This not only reduced the smell, but more importantly killed the "endoza" (another term for describing the micro-world they were discovering) which normally infected livestock. Another revolutionary discovery for health which originated from an interconnection (in this case logical, substantial, and interdisciplinary) which proved its circularity.

So, what did Lister do?

He figured that if disinfection could protect animals, why wouldn't it work in people? He made the surgeons in his ward wash their hands with an antiseptic soap (initially containing phenol). This intuition came after noticing that a phenolic solution immediately stopped an infection when it was applied to medicate a cut. He then started to apply it to clothing, patients and their wounds, dramatically decreasing the rate of mortal post-operative infections. Another one of Lister's ideas was to require surgeons to wear latex gloves, rather than gloves made from porous materials. (In those days, doctors would often keep the same pair of cotton gloves on to examine several patients in the same day.) Finally, he introduced hygiene and disinfection procedures in operating theaters, which was one of the critical control points for microbial infection. These approaches mirror those implemented today in the face of multiple drug-resistant bacterial infections and viral infections.

How is it that no one thought of this sooner?

In those days they were fumbling around in the dark, even conceptually speaking. Today we tend to forget the revolutionary scope of ideas and procedures which are apparently basic or seem obvious, but which actually took decades to be accepted and established as standards. In this case, Lister went even further than the most advanced knowledge of his day. He was not particularly interested in knowing how to grow, or in isolating and classifying microbes, which was the primary scientific focus at that time. Instead, he proceeded like a knight on a chess board. Two steps forward, and then either one step to the left or right. He didn't move in a simple straight line.

He wanted to answer a question which in hindsight appears obvious: How can you kill microbes, or at least stop their proliferation, whatever their name and surname? In other words, is there a substance that can kill microbes, be they *E. coli* or *V. cholerae*? A basic, pragmatic question, but one which in itself was a great leap forward.

The procedures developed by Lister weren't immediately popular, though. At first, almost all his fellow surgeons opposed him. No one likes to change their habits, and there was very little understanding of the importance of hygiene and sterilization practices. To be fair, surgeons and nurses had a point: phenol is irritating to the eyes and mucous membranes in the nose, and it has a very unpleasant, pungent odor. These far from trivial characteristics hampered the immediate and extensive use of phenol. But only a few years later it would become impossible –

even unethical – to ignore the enormous benefits of introducing this type of disinfection. Lister's method would spread throughout hospitals in Europe, and was soon followed by a dramatic upsurge in post-infection and post-surgery survival rates. This closed yet another circle, paving the way for modern surgery.

At the time, what was the relationship between disease and microbes thought to be?

The link between microbes and disease was a primary focus of Koch's research, a question which he devoted the greater part of his career to. Perhaps his most influential work was developing the so-called "Koch's postulates." These were a sort of reasoned dogma, an interlocking mechanism based on logic. The bottom line here was the hypothesis that microbes could cause diseases, and that this mechanism could be recreated under laboratory conditions. This facilitated the true birth of experimental pathology.

So, Koch discovered the link between microbes and disease, while Snow and Lister developed preventive procedures for avoiding disease spread just as – in some respects – vaccines did. And what happened if someone had already contracted an infection?

That brings us to another key innovation and the issue of antibiotic therapies, which became a priority with the outbreak of World War I. In those days soldiers on the Western Front died more often from the complications of an infected wound than from actual combat. Given that war infections had many commonalities, there was a frantic effort to try to identify a substance capable of curing fatal infections. Particularly interested in this question was a Scottish bacteriologist who had been sent to the laboratories of a French military hospital on the Strait of Dover, not far from Dunkirk. He attracted the attention of senior officers thanks to the reputation he'd gained in his private practice in London. To supplement his income, he would treat his famous and wealthy patients afflicted by syphilis (yes, the same disease which had inspired Fracastoro). His remedy was something new called salvarsan, which means "saved by arsenic." From this procedure, he realized that the same substance could be a solution for treating other infections too, like the ones they were seeing on the war front. We're obviously talking about Alexander Fleming (1881–1955): another man who knew how to look further afield, even beyond the scope of his own personal discoveries.

The father of penicillin.

Rather than the "father of the scientific community," we could refer to him as the talent-scout of antibiotics. Alexander Fleming was the seventh of eight children; his father died when he was young. Prior to studying medicine, he had enlisted in the Scottish army and fought in the Boer War. An ambitious student, in 1906 he was admitted to the Inoculation Department at St. Mary Hospital, an institution established only a few years before by Almroth Wright (1861–1947), the famed bacteriologist who had discovered a vaccine for typhoid fever.

With the outbreak of World War I, Wright was appointed colonel and sent to France to set up a laboratory and research center at Boulogne-sur-Mer, taking Fleming with him. The work that lay ahead of them was of titanic proportions as they had to deal with wounded soldiers in a hospital under war conditions. The only remedies available were carbolic acid, boric acid, and hydrogen peroxide; these substances were better than nothing, but they had side-effects and limitations. There was still a missing element: the cure. Fleming was determined to find it.

Clearly, he succeeded, despite the challenges.

Yes, but not immediately. At the end of the war Fleming resumed his work at St. Mary's, dedicating his efforts to the search for drugs that could fight bacteria. He was really committed, and quite creative too. One day when he was sick with a terrible cold, he added a drop of his mucus to a bacterial culture: to his total surprise he observed that the bacteria very quickly died. He had just discovered lysozyme, one of our natural defenses against infection (which unfortunately couldn't be repurposed as a drug). A dead end on his journey. The year was 1922.

But he persevered.

He certainly did! Six years later, in the summer, Fleming began studying staphylococcus bacteria. These are terrible germs, capable of provoking a number of dangerous infections (in the urinary tract, in the lungs and on the skin). One day Fleming inoculated some petri dishes with a staphylococcus culture, forgot it on his work bench and then went off for a two-week holiday.[1]

I can imagine Fleming's surprise when he got back...

It's not clear how, but two things occurred by an amazing coincidence: the first was that some mold spores had accidently made their way into the petri dish containing the bacterial culture. And that's plausible, as it has happened to most bacteriologists at some point in their careers. It also seems that on the ground floor of the same building another scientist was working on fungal cultures, keeping windows and doors wide-open... which explains how the right mold landed in the right petri dish. What's more curious though is that Fleming had forgotten the culture outside the incubator. So, the petri dishes in his experiment remained on the lab bench for two weeks at a room temperature of 25°C, conditions which allow both staphylococcus and mold to grow. To be clear, nothing would have happened had the petri dish been incubated at 37°C, or had it been put in the refrigerator. This discovery was the result of a unique series of accidental circumstances.

When you put it that way, the coincidence is truly striking.

If four different drivers hadn't coincided – the growth of bacteria, the growth of the mold, the right temperature and a two-week holiday – Fleming wouldn't have seen anything, and the hidden secret wouldn't have been revealed. Instead, when he got back and looked at the culture, he immediately noticed that, just like an egg white surrounding the yolk, there was a ring of clear agar around the mold, free of bacteria. A real miracle! Where had Mother Nature hidden some of its most potent molecules to combat epidemics and pestilence? Puerperal fevers after childbirth and septicemia? Pneumonia, nephritis and gastroenteritis? Basically everything from an abscessed tooth to infections from battle wounds? In molds! The miraculous mold was initially identified as *Penicillium rubrum* (although two years later it was discovered that in fact it was *Penicillium notatum*): hence the name Penicillin.

Lucky scientist, I would say.

It was actually Pasteur who once said, "Chance favors only the prepared mind." In the history of science, only a few people could embody this better than Fleming. In any event, as we've seen, luck helped many of our revolutionaries.

But now there's a question for all of us to consider. With the exception of Lady Mary Wortley Montagu, we've only been talking about men. To make amends for that obvious imbalance, it's important to mention an outstanding woman who fled Italy to escape from the racial laws promulgated by the fascist regime in the 1930s, who became a successful researcher in the United States, who established research institutes in Italy, won a Nobel Prize and became a Senator for Life of the Italian Republic. I'm talking about Rita Levi-Montalcini (1909–2012). Along with Stanley Cohen (1909–2020), she discovered Nerve Growth Factor (NGF), the first of a long list of substances which are now known to stimulate nerve growth. And just as antibiotics for fighting fevers and disease lay hidden in molds, nerve growth factor was hidden in snake venom. You heard me: *snake venom*! They might as well have found it in a dinosaur egg! But what is NGF? This substance makes it possible to regenerate nerve cells, the ones found in the brain and the spinal cord, which allow us to think, move, and perceive touch. Not only did Rita Levi-Montalcini and Stanley Cohen discover what NGF did, they also identified a source, which would enable them and others to study it in greater depth.

In this long journey, where we mainly rode on the back of microscopic creatures (so familiar to the people who work in the field), the story of Rita Levi-Montalcini brings us another connection: the connection with other disciplines. The astonishing presence of a growth factor for nerve cells in snake venom is only one example of the "improbable interconnections" which have paved the way to today's health standards. No doubt, an oncologist would give you a similar narrative. Maybe, with different characters, but essentially based on the discoveries in animals which led to studies on oncogenic viruses and investigations into the environment's role as a risk factor for many forms of cancer. A path to awareness which has branched out in multiple directions, enabling us to understand certain transversal mechanisms.

Let's return briefly to infectious diseases. With prevention, vaccines, and antibiotics, we have almost everything. Can we start declaring victory?

Not if on the other side you have the power of nature, and its incredible, vigorous resilience. This is the reason that a revolutionary such as Fleming surpassed himself with such clear vision and foresight. In an interview given in 1945, fresh from receiving the Nobel Prize for medicine, he said very likely sooner or later bacteria would become resistant to antibiotics, and he warned doctors and researchers against abusing these drugs. Just ten years after penicillin started being used on a global scale, some initial evidence of antibiotic resistance had already emerged. Today, less than a century after the discovery of antibiotics, the problem of super-killer bacteria risks overwhelming us. And this could be the best possible motivation to open the discussion on circular and interconnected health, in today's digital world.

Notes

[1] The Petri dish is a basic tool in numerous areas of biology used to grow cell cultures; it allows us to observe bacterial colonies with the naked eye. The name comes from the man who invented it in 1877, the bacteriologist Julius Richard Petri (1852–1921), one of Robert Koch's assistants. The most common petri dishes have a diameter between 50 and 100mm, and are 15mm high.

0   A New Way Forward

We're coming to the end of this conversation, and I'd like to go back to the question we started with: what's wrong with the way we see Health today?

In many parts of the planet we've attained levels of Health which would have been unthinkable just a few years ago. At the same time there are many signs indicating that humans as a species are encountering threats that are potentially existential. We're facing enormous challenges, such as extending the well-being we currently enjoy in the West to other countries in a way that's compatible with our planet's existing resources. It's becoming obvious that the system we're currently operating with is broken. Until now, human beings have taken charge of the planet's well-being. Some things have worked well; others haven't. To be honest, we've mismanaged some resources so badly we've come to the point of contending that some changes may prove insurmountable if we don't take corrective action soon. What's certain is that we need an innovative approach that will enable us to move health forward to become a comprehensive, inclusive system. To do this, we must develop new, fully interdisciplinary areas of research that will allow us to go beyond the established way of doing things. In such a demanding moment, we should be laying the groundwork and creating the infrastructure for a new paradigm.

How can we do this?

By changing our mindset and leveraging the opportunities available today, some that would have been inconceivable in the past.

For example, by taking advantage of an extraordinary phenom-enon at this point in history, the dawn of a new dimension: big data.

Do we have to join the group of intellectuals today who are obsessed with big data?

It's becoming the reality we live in. Consider some numbers: in 2017 a computer prototype was developed capable of simultane-ously managing 160 terabytes of data – an amount equal to five times the information contained in all the volumes of the Library of Congress in Washington DC (the largest library in the world – processed by a single machine)! In 2018, more than 3 million gigabytes of Internet traffic per minute were used in the United States alone. If we trust future predictions, in less than five years, 150 billion devices will be online – that's 20 times the world's population!

A frightening number...

...which is growing exponentially. Just think, the volume of information churned out in 2016 alone was equal to the total amount of data produced in the entire history of humankind, all years combined, up to 2015. And how long will it take for that amount of information to double within the next ten years? The prediction is truly stunning: 12 hours! Yes, every 12 hours the volume of data generated globally will double.

And what are we going to do with this infinite amount of in-formation?

Many things. Today, information about a lot of our activities is already collected, analyzed and "used" in real time. And we can already take pictures of foods in restaurants and supermar-kets with our smart phones and immediately find out what in-gredients they contain, as well as nutrients and calories. Tech-nology is rapidly becoming more and more wearable too, allow-ing us to not only measure vital statistics such as heart rate and blood pressure but also to get a daily digital snapshot of where, what, when and how much we've eaten, drunk, walked and slept. We can track many other functions as well, physiological or not. In the parallel digital dimension, we each already have a growing number of avatars, our doubles, made up only of data. We're all becoming clouds, evolving data bundles. Have you ever seen a digital alarm clock that projects the time on the ceiling? Well, just think of this: we ourselves have become "data generators" that are projected elsewhere. And there, inside one or more servers, which are not necessarily located in the same place, lies the projection(s) of our existence, in digital format.

That doesn't sound very reassuring...

And it doesn't just concern humans – but also animals, plants and the environment. Our cultivated land and livestock are digitalized as well, and for years we've been measuring environmental variables such as temperature, humidity, pollen count and UV radiation – as well as hurricane intensity, the oceans heating and the ice caps melting. For years now we've mapped the migration of insects, the proliferation of invasive species and the spread of infectious diseases. A maddening exercise of classifying, recording and accumulating facts... oftentimes with clearly defined experimental end points.

How will the new technologies change the way we relate to the environment?

In the past we would only separate red apples from yellow, making a note of their weight when we handpicked them and placed them in crates. Nowadays we're able to track the progress of every single apple, from when it's a flower to when it becomes a fruit all the way to when it turns into jam: nutritional value, origin, size, weight, species and variety. All in real time. We'll understand new things as we record reality frame by frame. This is where we'll gain extraordinary insights and we'll have a chance to establish a more integrated and respectful relationship with the environment around us.

Surely we will need an inconceivable amount of processing power to analyze all this data.

Yes that's right. The other opportunity, in addition to big data, is artificial intelligence and computing power. And major multinational corporations are realizing this and investing. As an example, IBM has launched a project called "Watson Health." It's not a reference to Sherlock Holmes's assistant (although it could be) but to Thomas J. Watson, IBM's first president. For this project, a computer has "learned" more than 35 million research papers in all areas of medical science, assimilated an enormous amount of real clinical data. And based on a grid of symptoms and information on the patient, this machine can provide diagnostic recommendations to physicians. We don't realize it yet, but what we have before us is a vast range of incredible opportunities. Soon we'll be able to feed our entire clinical history into a machine and our doctors will get potential diagnostic scenarios for our clinical problem. Each one of us will eventually benefit from a full electronic health record which would contain our medical records and additional information on the components of health: our diet, our physical exercise, how much water or alcohol we drink. But if we follow the lead of John Snow and his groundbreaking work on cholera, we'd also include where we live and where we source our food and water. And so on...

Can Artificial Intelligence and big data really revolutionize our concept of health?

All the health revolutionaries we've mentioned here swam against the current, questioning the prevailing theories of their time. What's more, they confronted enormous obstacles because they didn't have access to information or the real-time communications mechanisms we have today. In effect, they pulled down walls, one brick at a time, with their bare hands. One of their challenges was collecting the information they needed without any support system, and for this feat alone they deserve our respect and admiration. Today the situation is completely different: we are immersed in information – big data – but we are actually a bit afraid of it. We don't see the immense potential it holds for society as a whole.

Can you give me an example of how big data could be used to advance scientific progress?

Our mobile devices work like antennas that detect and transmit data in real time, which is something we are only partially aware of. The revolutionary thinkers of the past had to draw by hand, now we take photographs. And while only a few of us can draw well, and accurately represent reality (think of the drawings by Vesalius or Leonardo Da Vinci), we're all more or less capable of taking a photo. To oversimplify, let's look at the positive side of technology: in theory, compared to what we were only a century ago, today we are clearly superheroes. Today we move faster than the speed of sound – forget travelling by horseback, trying to avoid plague outbreaks and ambushes. We don't have to do calculations because someone taught a machine to do them for us (the simple calculator). If the revolutionary minds we mentioned earlier could have benefited from the tools we have today, their discoveries wouldn't have taken so many centuries. Technology definitely provides some incredible opportunities; even though it's not enough on its own.

So what's missing?

First and most importantly, awareness. The gist of this argument is that if we acknowledge that health is a universal asset, and if we agree on the interconnections and interdependences that pertain to it, we can't continue doing what we're doing. We can't continue polluting, invading, abusing either deliberately, accidentally or carelessly, as if the environment were our exclusive property and ecosystems didn't really matter. We're out of excuses.

We must adopt a new vision and new behaviors, at all levels. Just think that in many advanced countries, people blithely throw their unused medicines into household trash, along with batteries and electronic devices. This may sound like a cliché, but we can't keep on wrecking our own home. We can't trash it, tear it down and then expect to suffer no consequences, either for ourselves or our housemates.

But Mother Nature is resilient, that we know.

Then let's talk about a massive problem: the erosion of biodiversity. Biodiversity is not just about the extinction of the Pangolin. This scaled mammal (take a look at it) is ruthlessly hunted for its flesh and its scales, which are used in traditional Chinese medicine. (A little while ago a stash of scales was found from approximately 10,000 pangolins.) Or the disappearance of cheetahs and African wild dogs. Or rhinos, massacred for their horns. Biodiversity is much more than these atrocious examples. Biodiversity is the elasticity of life on Earth, the capacity to absorb disturbance in the face of slow or rapid change. If a cold snap arrives, maybe a plant will survive because it's different from the rest. Because it's different. Maintaining diversity is key.

If all the elements of a living system are genetically identical, none of them will survive a catastrophe that might strike that species. If, on the other hand, they differ from one another in some way, then perhaps one or two genotypes will survive. And adding to the importance of biodiversity, today we are looking for painkillers in the venom of marine creatures, and new drugs or antibiotics in the most improbable creatures. Diversity counts. If these species disappear, reserves of special molecules – whether known or unknown to us today – will disappear too. For all we know, Mother Nature probably hid some miraculous molecule in the antenna of the Borneo moth. We just need to find it.

The most recent United Nations report is clear as far as the major engines that are bulldozing their way through biodiversity. The unregulated over-utilization of land and sea. The excessive exploitation of living organisms, climate change, pollution and invasive species.

In other words, the data suggest that we're the ones who should do something about it?

Humans are the self-appointed dominant species; we hold the key to the system, and that is a huge responsibility. Let's stop and think for a minute: whether we like it or not, human beings are capable of understanding certain mechanisms and acting on them. No other species has this ability. An earthworm certainly can't be expected to care about circular health (even though it impacts everyday life for organisms that live naked and underground), or an artichoke or a starfish for that matter. Can the amazing spaceship we're happily hitching a ride on be expected to function if we demolish its engine and frame?

We all want a healthier planet, but what can we do about it?

To start with, instead of focusing only on health in a vertical, hyper-specialized way, we should go back to thinking more broadly, understanding the need for a wider perspective, and adopt more far-sighted policies. But we need to be careful because we've run out of excuses. We can't keep on looking the other way, and refuse to take the opportunity of understanding where we've gone wrong. Up to now we've behaved as if the reserves and resilience of the planet and its inhabitants were infinite. But that's not the case; mistakes have been made. Many, way too many. Today big data provide us with instruments for analyzing those mistakes, and understanding their impact and ramifications, offering an infinity of new opportunities to think in terms of circular health, while keeping a sharp focus on ethics.

So what lies ahead?

You can start thinking about the next phase when you've accomplished the goals of the previous one, either completely or partially, or when you've exhausted a particular approach. It looks like we've reached a level of verticality so deep that if we continue to hyper-specialize we risk not being able to use the infinite potential we have at our disposal today. Instead, we should be aiming at comprehensively responsible innovation.

The United Nations Sustainable Development Goals say the same thing. And in this regard let's not forget that responsible innovation also means optimizing resources and using what's already available.

Today we're going through a revolution which was inconceivable in the past. But in this new dimension, this Garden of Eden of numerals with hidden and forbidden meanings, it's absolutely essential that we all make an extra effort. Revolutionaries and change-makers must look to the future with a vision that includes responsibility.

Where could this new path take us with particular reference to medicine?

New technologies create new possibilities, empowering us to completely rethink the way we relate to health. And we have to come to terms with another group of people asking for change: patients. It's inevitable that their voices will become stronger and, let's hope, even more informed and aware. Patients can drive change by influencing the demand side of the equation in what is effectively a service industry: healthcare.

Do you mean that there also has to be a change in the relationship between scientists and the rest of the population, between doctors and patients?

We need to pay much more attention to the needs of the stakeholders (patients). But we can also benefit from tools that weren't available in the past, tools that can help us understand certain mechanisms. If someone calls, screaming and shouting from the sea of confusion that is the Internet, it means they want to open a dialogue. Today this can be done, so that the relationship with the patient becomes more active and bidirectional. This is a necessary step for everyone to achieve greater empowerment over their own health. That empowerment should allow us as a community to service the needs of the many whilst also servicing the needs of the few.

Returning to the issue of information, let's put ourselves in a researcher's shoes. How can you reconcile the staggering amount of studies, research and information on health into a single vision?

What has changed is that today we have the instruments we need to do this. The sources of information multiply with the launch of every new model of our inseparable measuring sticks – smart phones, cars, household appliances, thermostats, and sensors – they're everywhere: in homes, factories and farms. In addition to this "passive" recording mode, there is also a more active one, which concerns for instance the participation in data collection.

And it's not just a question of technology. In addition to the Internet and big data, there's another dimension we have overlooked, and we tend to take for granted today: globalization. Discovery very often originates from a process of understanding and seizing opportunities beyond national borders (and mental boundaries).

There are certain constants in each of the stories we have recounted: one is that great discoveries are nurtured by different cultures, interpretations and points of view. Recall Vesalius – a Flemish man from Brussels, who taught at the University of Padua, published his masterpiece in Switzerland and then moved to the imperial court of Spain. The globalization of science is not a modern invention: scholars and researchers have always been global citizens.

Besides, if I'm not mistaken, you've always felt passionately about free circulation of scientific data.

The data-sharing movement that's happening now is the obvious continuation of a personal journey I began many years ago.

In 2006, when I was still working in Italy (at the "Istituto Zoo-profilattico delle Venezie" at Legnaro, near Padua), we decided to share the genetic sequence of an influenza virus in birds that we had just decoded, on an open-access platform available to all scientists. Before long, my initiative became known worldwide. I did receive some harsh criticism, but for the most part we received support and achieved the consensus of the scientific community.

Who else was involved then?

It was just the right time for a paradigm shift and several leading researchers realized this, joining the initiative. If the timing is right, the wave of change will turn into a storm surge. Ours was an intuition which landed on fertile ground, so to speak.

Did it create a lot of buzz?

Quite a bit. We found our team's work on the pages of the *New York Times* and the *Wall Street Journal*. It felt like we had landed in something way bigger than ourselves. But we were always confident that we'd made the right choice. At that time researchers worldwide needed more data and more genetic sequences. We made ours public and free, setting an example, and inviting others to do the same.

What did that experience teach you personally?

That sharing information is imperative, and everyone should do their part. As we've said earlier in this book, scientific progress has been limited over the years by researchers failing to do the right thing – sharing their findings – and doing it right away. Our initiative wouldn't have made any sense if it hadn't been taken up by many other researchers and organizations, promoting the philosophy and culture of open access. One more genetic sequence doesn't change much, but thousands of sequences allow you to delve deeper. So, really, our ultimate goal was achieved by the scientific community, not just by a single scientist.

And what can ordinary folks, kids, parents, retired people do in such a large-scale initiative?

We just talked about data being collected passively, or "retrieved," and actively-generated: information about health and vital statistics, such as blood pressure and glycemic index, eating and exercise habits, can be combined with environmental data such as pollution levels. Information of this kind could play an essential role in understanding the long-term effects of certain substances and drugs, for example. Today these kinds of studies are very expensive and take years to complete, but with a paradigm shift, knowledge on these topics could get a huge boost. Digital epidemiology is already here, it's just waiting to release its full potential.

Epidemiologists look for signs, recent or ancient, left by a disease or an infection. The tracks we've studied up till now were more or less like footprints left by bare feet on the sand: there's not much to observe or measure, more or less just length and width. But the tracks we can analyze today are more like the detailed prints left by a soccer boot on wet sand, with its studs and the writing on the outer sole. A 3D printout, as it were, with a lot of additional information. So we can say that up to now we've only studied a small, specific part of the problem.

Why should we consent to sharing our data: isn't it a bit like being a guinea pig?

Essentially, data-sharing is better for all of us. There are still so many things that we don't know about physiological or pathological mechanisms. So by activating participatory processes that leverage big data, we could truly give incredible impetus to the study of certain pathologies, starting with cancer and diabetes, which would in turn lead to the development of therapies. It's also an issue of social responsibility: if we all move in the same direction with greater awareness we may be able to trigger a series of positive spirals.

Can you explain this better?

We could set in motion an acceleration of the kind of research that requires a massive quantity of data on biological, physical, biochemical and behavioral parameters. This would provide countless opportunities in health care: data would allow us to connect many dots. But for most scientists, big data are an opportunity to advance their own field of research as opposed to representing a resource for the cross-sectional advance of health as a system. Of course it's necessary to keep making progress in individual fields, and follow our tracks; but now the time has come to look at things from another perspective, maybe even an NL one.

NL? The Dutch again?

The Dutch have nothing to do with being NL (even if there are many NLs among the Dutch, starting with van Leeuwenhoek). I have come this far to propose that a reasoned and interdisciplinary use of big data could lead us to a broader vision, which embraces health in all its facets. For example, let's think about the treatment of depression or neurodegenerative diseases, a very complex and rather novel field of health. Mental diseases, until a few decades ago, weren't even considered true diseases. Gradually, the therapeutic focus shifted towards pharmacological interventions, and now more and more studies are broadening their scope to look at other factors that may cause these pathologies, including personal or family relations.

For more specifics, today we're experimenting with enhanced environments for Alzheimer patients – working with interior decorators and designers to provide them with more stimulating surroundings. And again along the lines of sensory stimulation, the Mayo Clinic recognizes the benefits of music for patients with Alzheimer or dementia. Science tells us that the parts of the brain involved in musical memory are relatively unaffected compared to other parts in patients with these specific pathologies – so by evoking musical memories, stress, anxiety and depression can be reduced.

Treatments with music and colored light-bulbs? Aren't we slipping into a New Age approach? We already have people offering treatment based on listening or empathy, or chili and lemons…

Oh no! That approach can be extremely dangerous. Let's set things straight: science is science and it concerns itself with what is quantifiable and measurable, what can be verified. Falsifiable evidence and claims, to quote Karl Popper. But it's true that today, with new data, we can study phenomena which were much harder to observe and measure in the past, at the intersection between biology and social behavior.

Let's get back to the point: do we necessarily have to accept being under scrutiny every second of our lives for the sake of scientific progress?

In our society at present, this is already how things work. Weren't you texting on your phone just a few minutes ago? Haven't you checked your emails today or bought something online? Haven't you used your credit card or browser? Haven't you played a game on your smart phone, or liked or shared a post on a social network? Today we're already handing out our data left and right: it would certainly make more sense to use these data anonymously for a good cause, for everyone's benefit. Technology is now a part of us; it's a prosthesis we interact with: why not transform all of this into positive energy, something which can benefit collective knowledge and wellbeing?

So you think that privacy isn't an issue?

It's a very serious issue, and it has to be dealt with by experts. But there's nothing wrong with speculating on new scenarios, while legal experts and computer scientists work on finding a balance between opposing needs.

Do you believe that it will be possible to arrive at a concept of health as a circular equilibrium of human-animal-plant-environment?

The idea we should all consider is that we can't keep thinking of human health as our sole primary objective, whether as individuals or as a species. We must manage health as a system. Our forecasting capacity is growing at a dizzying pace: in this scenario, for example, we can no longer study malaria or Zika while ignoring global warming. Ultimately, a core component of knowledge is identifying connections between things and information, and today we can cross-check and analyze a mushrooming amount of data. Again, take Zika for instance: did you know a huge impact on the spread of the epidemic came from the flow of tourists and cruise ships? Epidemiologists were able to identify proliferation patterns by looking at shipping routes. This is where the "rubber" of big data really "hits the road."

Where do mistakes in managing the human-animal-environment interactions really impact us?

Fleming had foreseen it, and now we have reached the critical point he feared. The Scottish scientist had predicted that "intelligent bacteria" would learn to resist antibiotics, and, sure enough, the abuse of antibiotics has resulted in super-killer bacteria. To make matters worse, antibiotics have been used systematically even in livestock, resulting in the selection and circulation of super-resistant bacteria. We really should have seen that coming...

What do you mean by circulation?

Cow bacteria aren't confined to cows. Quite the opposite: mechanisms of food production and distribution can bring to our table microbes that should definitely not be there. Just think that towards the end of 2018, a contamination of *Escherichia coli* O157:H7 from a batch of infected lettuce affected sixteen US states. Sixteen. The contaminated lettuce not only ended up on supermarket shelves but also in large-scale sandwich production. And where do you think this specific strain of bacteria came from? To put it delicately, from the intestines of cows, sheep, and deer. And from there, how did the microbes get onto the lettuce in sixteen different states? Through field fertigation (the injection of fertilizers into irrigation systems), and then via distribution chains – with trucks delivering produce right to our kitchens. *E. coli* is a food-borne bacterium that liberates toxins which can have severe consequences, including disability or death. It makes its way to our kitchen and antibiotics are completely useless.

In short, we've developed production mechanisms that are completely vertical.

And they could be called selfish. If we upset ecological and natural mechanisms to boost productivity, we have to remember that the cost-benefit analysis doesn't only concern the present, but mostly the future, in the middle- and long-term.

In the world of companion animals, for example, let's say our best friend – our dog – gets cancer treatment in the form of chemotherapy, which manages to lengthen the life of our pet by a few months. Aside from any specific considerations, in addition to chemotherapy these "patients" end up needing repeated rounds of antibiotics, just as humans do, because chemotherapy makes them immune-suppressed and weak. And guess what happens? Their feces contain an extremely high percentage of multi-drug resistant bacteria. From this we can draw the conclusion that fragile human patients run an especially high risk of contracting infections which will then be very difficult to treat.

It is essential to underline that we know the mechanisms, paths and dangers involved here. We can no longer say "it is not my problem." We function as a community, not as individuals; the actions of every single person indirectly affect the lives of everybody else, not only in pandemics.

By the way, lately we've heard a lot about vaccinations and, more particularly, about the anti-vax movement.

It might not be appropriate to get into specific national situations, so let's look at the purpose of the anti-vax movement instead. In general, they want to transform the population from "resistant" to "receptive" with regard to microbes that we've learned how to fight through vaccinations. Some anti-vaxxers may say that this isn't their primary goal, but it is clearly the functional consequence of their belief. And if they achieve this, we would be taking one step forward and one step back. The step back would be that average life expectancy would drop drastically. Once the new system becomes "operational" so to speak, new generations would be totally unprotected from chicken pox, the measles, whooping cough, and tetanus, which would claim victims on a large scale. The leading cause of death would become infectious diseases and their complications. Many more would get sick, develop fevers and blisters, and would be unable to leave the house.

And what would the step forward be in this ominous scenario?

It could be said, to play the devil's advocate, that such a marked decline in life expectancy (which may even drop as low as 60!), would lead to a radical resolution of all issues tied to public health expenses and pensions. But I doubt that anyone (even the anti-vaxxers) would see such a catastrophe as a real advantage for society.

That sounds drastic. But let's get back to the issue of individual and collective good.

It's clear that there are parallel paths to the ones we've set off on so far. The revolutionary people in this book (all men except for two women, sadly) searched for real innovation by challenging dogmas and widening their field vision to embrace other disciplines. Today we could use the immense amount of information generated for different purposes and continue that spirit of scientific discovery, finding something that is at the limit of conceivability: being non-lateralized.

Not lateralized… is that what NL means?

Yes! To simplify, let's say that a small percentage of the population cannot distinguish left from right – relative to themselves, and consequently to the world around them. The process of left-right discrimination (here referred to as lateralization[1]) occurs around the first year of primary school, and if you miss that window of awareness, left and right will never have meaning for you. This means that non-lateralized people are unable to follow directions such as "first go right, then take the second on your left." They frequently get lost, often going down the wrong corridor or alley. At the same time, the non-lateralized person knows that left and right are only a representation: they are a conjecture and not an intrinsic characteristic of reality, even though this seems to be the case for everyone else.

Are you suggesting a "non-lateralized" approach to the challenges we've talked about? Without prejudices, but also without reference points?

Well, perhaps the first lesson we should remember in order to allow health to advance as a system, is to leave the main road and reclaim the courage and candor which characterized the people we've spoken of.

Everyone should occasionally try to adopt the non-lateralized perspective, by looking beyond the physical and mental boundaries imposed on us. Left and right are useful, but at times – in interstellar space, for instance – they just create confusion.

The real key to reading the future is to use new languages to communicate science, as Vesalius did, and have the courage to challenge established beliefs with the unthinkable, like Fracastoro did. In other words, we have to discover the new invisible parallel worlds which influence our health, and make these worlds accessible.

We should look at the opportunities we have, without pre-conceived ideas. Is this your message?

This book tells of a journey through time. It is a story of people, ideas, and concepts seen through an interdisciplinary lens. Throughout the centuries, "re-shuffling the cards" has often led to revolutionary transformations: this observation cannot be denied. Constant reshuffling fuels growth and curiosity. If it happens by chance it cannot be controlled. However, it is possible to deliberately map out structured paths to empower what, today, is known as disruptive innovation.

The time is right for this transformation. Big data is out there waiting for us. All we need is to believe in interdisciplinarity: history teaches us that a multi-stakeholder perspective makes great discoveries possible and this can enable us to transform health from a small homo-centric pillar to a large multi-dimensional sphere.

Looking for new points of reference is always useful but at times, it is critical.

If it's a matter of Health, it's absolutely vital.

Notes

[1] In Italian, a confusion or difficulty with left-right discrimination may be defined as *non lateralizzato* and is referred to in the original text as NL. This wording and acronym thus creates a narrative curiosity that features centrally in subsequent discussions throughout the treatise. For the sake of clarity, the term *lateralization* when referring to brain functions, has a very specific meaning. It defines abilities or functions that are disproportionately focused to one side of the brain. A clear example of this is language, which localizes for the most part on the left hemisphere. For narrative purposes the acronym NL has been maintained in this English version.

Bibliography

G. Armocida, B. Zanobio, *Storia della Medicina*, Milano, Masson, 2003.

L. Bertinato, «Mediterranean routes and the bulwarks of plague control during the "Serenissima Republic" in Venice», *World Neurology*, 30 January 2017.

F. Bottacciolo, *Filosofia per la medicina, medicina per la filosofia. Grecia e Cina a confronto*, Milano, Tecniche Nuove, 2010.

V. Boudon-Millot, *Galeno di Pergamo: un medico greco a Roma*, Roma, Carocci, 2016.

W.A.C. Bullock, A. Fleming, *The Man Who Discovered Penicillin. A Life of Sir Alexander Fleming*, London, Faber & Faber, 1963.

G. Canguilhem, *Le normal et le pathologique*, Paris, Puf, 1966.

W.R. Clark, *At War Within: The Double-Edged Sword of Immunity*, New York, Oxford University Press, 1995.

L.I. Conrad, Cambridge University Press, *The Western Medical Tradition: 800 B.C. to A.D. 1800*, Cambridge, Cambridge University Press, 2011.

G. Cosmacini, *Medicina e sanità in Italia nel ventesimo secolo: dalla "spagnola" alla II guerra mondiale*, Roma-Bari, Laterza, 1989.

G. Cosmacini, *L'arte lunga. Storia della medicina dall'antichità a oggi*, Roma-Bari, Laterza, 2011.

G. Cosmacini, C. Crisciani, *Medicina e filosofia nella tradizione dell'Occidente*, Milano, Episteme Edizioni, 1998.

G. Cosmacini, M. Menghi, V. Boudon-Millot, *Galeno e il galenismo: Scienza e idee della salute*, Milano, FrancoAngeli, 2012.

U. Curi, *Le parole della cura. Medicina e filosofia*, Milano, Raffaello Cortina, 2017.

U. Eco, *Sulle spalle dei giganti: Lezioni alla Milanesiana, 2001-2015*, Milano, La nave di Teseo, 2017.

Galeno, M. Vegetti, *Nuovi scritti autobiografici*, Roma, Carocci, 2013.

Galeno, M. Vegetti, I. Garofalo, *Opere scelte di Galeno*, Torino, Utet, 1978.

S. Giardina, A.G. Spagnolo, «Le virtù della storia: la sfida tra dogma e innovazione nella rivoluzione anatomica di Andrea Vesalio», *Biografie Mediche*, 2013 (2), pp. 7-9.

D. Helbing *et al.*, «Will democracy survive big data and artificial intelligence?», *Scientific American*, 25 February 2017.

S. Hempel, *The Strange Case of the Broad Street Pump: John Snow and the Mystery of Cholera*, Berkeley, University of California Press, 2007.

R.D. Huerta, J. Vermeer, *Giants of Delft: Johannes Vermeer and the Natural Philosophers: The Parallel Search for Knowledge During the Age of Discovery*, Lewisburg, Bucknell University Press, 2003.

Ippocrate, M. Vegetti, *Opere di Ippocrate*, Torino, Utet, 2000.

H. King, *Health in Antiquity*, London, Routledge, 2005.

I. Loudon, Oxford University Press, *Western Medicine: An Illustrated History*, Oxford, Oxford University Press, 2005.

V. Nutton, *Ancient Medicine*, London, Routledge, 2014.

R. Porter, *Blood and Guts: A Short History of Medicine*, New York, W.W. Norton, 2003.

Storia del pensiero medico occidentale, edited by M. Grmek, voll. 3, Roma-Bari, Laterza, 1993-1998.

A. Touwaide, *Medical Traditions*, Berlin, De Gruyter, 2020.

F. Zampieri, *Storia della medicina dalla preistoria ai nostri giorni*, Padova, Cleup, 2016.

A. Vesalius, V. Nutton, *Principles of Anatomy According to the Opinion of Galen by Johann Guinter and Andreas Vesalius*, Basingstoke, Taylor & Francis, 2017.

Acknowledgments

My heartfelt thanks go to all those who supported me, each in their own way, in this bizarre but ambitious conceptual project. I'm not just referring to Beppe Ippolito, Ilaria Borletti Buitoni, Mario Rasetti, Giovanna Guzzetti, Sergio Saia, Eligio Piccolo – if you were there to back me up in this atypical enterprise, I really thank you.

I would like to thank Cristina Alberini, Professor at the Center for Neural Science at New York University, for helping me disentangle the term "lateralization" from the traps that writing in two languages can generate.

But I owe a special thanks to two people.

The first one goes to Umberto Curi, for being the one who made philosophy approachable to me. An essential step in my life, which helped me push my own mental boundaries.

And then a special thank-you to Sara Agnelli. I strongly wanted a classicist in my working group at the University of Florida. Being exposed to the world of classics I have learned to appreciate the role of disruptive innovators of the past in leveraging knowledge to gain the health we have today. I believe that as people who operate in science, we have an obligation to look back from time to time.

If only for the perspective, compared to the micro-micro-micro detail we're dealing with.

Contributors

Sara Agnelli graduated in Classical Literature from the Catholic University of Milan. After receiving a Ph.D. in Classics from the University of Florida, in 2017, she started working at the One Health Center of Excellence, where she's been responsible for interdisciplinary relations between the Sciences and the Humanities.

Daniele Mont D'Arpizio lives and works in Padua. Journalist and writer, he focuses mainly on science, culture, and history.

Alberto Fioretti graduated in Philosophy at the Sapienza University of Rome.